CARING FOR THE WORLD:
A GUIDEBOOK TO GLOBAL HEALTH OPPORTUNITIES

As disparities in health care continue to widen between wealthy and impoverished nations, an increasing number of medical professionals are committing themselves to the growing field of global health. *Caring for the World* assembles the stories, experience, and advice of prominent global health practitioners in this inspired guidebook for health care workers who are interested in – or already are – improving the lives of people throughout the world.

Providing a wealth of valuable resources and information, the authors detail how individuals can find and prepare for global health work as well as how to obtain education and funding from governmental and non-governmental organizations. Skilfully addressing important issues related to working within other countries and cultures, they also provide practical advice on how to understand pandemics and the HIV/AIDS crisis in order to effect change.

Accessible, thorough, and concise, *Caring for the World* is essential reading for anyone interested in global health work, non-governmental organizations, and the current state of global health care.

PAUL K. DRAIN is a resident physician at Stanford University Hospital.

STEPHEN A. HUFFMAN is the medical director of St Rita's Putnam County Emergency Room.

SARA E. PIRTLE is the coordinator of International Studies & Programs at the University of Nebraska Medical Center.

KEVIN CHAN is a fellow in the Munk Centre for International Studies and Centre for International Health at the University of Toronto.

PAUL K. DRAIN, STEPHEN A. HUFFMAN,
SARA E. PIRTLE, AND KEVIN CHAN

Caring for the World:

A Guidebook to Global Health Opportunities

UNIVERSITY OF TORONTO PRESS
Toronto Buffalo London

© University of Toronto Press Incorporated 2009
Toronto Buffalo London
www.utppublishing.com
Printed in Canada

ISBN 978-0-8020-9804-7 (cloth)
ISBN 978-0-8020-9548-0 (paper)

Printed on acid-free paper

Library and Archives Canada Cataloguing in Publication

Caring for the world : a guidebook to global health opportunities / Paul
K. Drain ... [et al.].

Includes index.
ISBN 978-0-8020-9804-7 (bound). – ISBN 978-0-8020-9548-0 (pbk.)

1. World health – Vocational guidance.   2. Medical personnel –
Employment – Foreign countries.   3. Medical assistance.   4. Public
health – International cooperation.   5. Voluntary health agencies.
6. Volunteer workers in medical care.   I. Drain, Paul K., 1974–

RA441.C37 2008   610.69   C2008-904576-9

University of Toronto Press acknowledges the financial assistance to its
publishing program of the Canada Council for the Arts and the Ontario
Arts Council.

University of Toronto Press acknowledges the financial support for its
publishing activities of the Government of Canada through the Book
Publishing Industry Development Program (BPIDP).

Health is a state of complete physical, mental and social well-being.

The enjoyment of the highest attainable standard of health is one of the fundamental rights of every human being without distinction of race, religion, political belief, economic or social condition.

The health of all peoples is fundamental to the attainment of peace and security and is dependent upon the fullest co-operation of individuals and States.

– Constitution of the World Health Organization,
adopted by the International Health Conference, July 1946

Contents

Authors' Note

Disparities in people's health and health care services between rich and poor countries have never been more profound. For the first time in history, according to recent World Health Organization statistics, the average life expectancy of people in one country (Japan, 82.2 years) is more than twice as long as the life expectancy of people in nine sub-Saharan African countries. In addition, the number of physicians per capita of one country (Cuba, 591 physicians per 100,000 people) is more than ten times the number of physicians per capita of seventy-one countries, and more than one hundred times the physicians per capita of fifteen countries. Finally, the average annual spending on health per person in the United States (U.S.$ 6,096) is greater than the amount of spending on health per person of the lowest seventy countries combined. In this era of technology and information, an infant born today in a 'developed country' is expected to live more than thirty years longer than an infant born in a 'developing country.'

These global disparities of health are unacceptable, and more action must be taken to improve the basic health and health services of people in poorer settings. Our primary aims in creating this guidebook are to facilitate a better understanding of global health issues and provide resources that help people become engaged in global health activities. This guidebook, which grew from our experiences of collecting and assimilating information on global health opportunities, is intended to serve as a comprehensive resource for any student or professional who seeks to become more engaged in the rapidly expanding field of global health and medicine. We intend for this guidebook to be useful for people with various educational backgrounds and all levels of global health experience.

As we encourage you to become more engaged, we hope that you do so with respect for the local communities. Being invited to participate in global health activities is a privilege, not a right. All people and societies, particularly those in a resource-poor setting, should be treated with a high level of respect for their culture, beliefs, religion, customs, and traditions.

The book is organized into four major sections. Chapters 1 and 2 provide an overview of global health and medicine, and describe some non-traditional pathways of becoming engaged in global health activities. The second section, comprised of chapters 3 through 7, serves as the main resource to the various programs, courses, conferences, organizations, academic opportunities, and funding available in global health and medicine. The third section, comprised solely of chapter 8, describes the logistical process of planning and preparing for a global health experience. Finally, chapters 9 and 10 present solicited advice from several leading global health experts, including Drs Allan Rosenfield, Richard Feachem, Jim Kim, Evaleen Jones, and Keith Brown, and conclude with some encouragement and suggestions for surviving and enjoying a global health experience.

As global health continues to rapidly expand and change, the information contained in this guidebook will become more outdated. We have made every attempt to provide accurate and comprehensive information. However, there will be some inaccuracies. The most up-to-date information should always be obtained by contacting the primary source, such as a funding agency or organization. Therefore, while we provide access to the information, you will need to verify its validity. If you do find inaccuracies or know of additional opportunities, then we would greatly appreciate hearing from you.

Finally, we thank you for becoming more engaged in global health. Collectively, we can reduce the global disparities of health and change the course of history.

Paul K. Drain, MD, MPH
Department of Medicine
Stanford University

Stephen A. Huffman, MD
Medical Director
St Rita's Putnam County Emergency Room
Premier Health Care Services
Tipp City, Ohio

Sara E. Pirtle, MBA
Coordinator of International Studies & Programs
University of Nebraska Medical Center

Kevin Chan, MD, MPH
Pediatric Emergency Physician
Hospital for Sick Children
Munk Centre for International Studies and
Centre for International Health
University of Toronto

Foreword

Interest in global health and resources for reducing disparities in global health have rapidly expanded during the past 20 years. Much of the growing interest has been driven by students and young professionals who seek to address global inequities, particularly inequities in availability and accessibility to health care resources. The current generation of students and young professionals continually seeks new educational and working opportunities in global health. These individuals are not only coming from the traditional pathways of public health, medicine, nursing, and anthropology, but now increasingly come from backgrounds in other health sciences, as well as economics, business, law, public affairs, education, engineering, bioengineering, urban planning, informatics, and many others. The interest and demand from these young professionals has helped shape a continually evolving field that will undoubtedly change the face of health care delivery and access around the world.

Before this guidebook, information had remained scattered among various websites, organizations, and lengthy textbooks. The authors of *Caring for the World: A Guidebook to Global Health Opportunities* have created a new, comprehensive resource for students, young professionals, administrators, and global health practitioners. They have collected a broad spectrum of information and compiled it in a format to readily assist anyone seeking to become more engaged in global health and medicine. This guidebook is comprehensive and timely, and will aid anyone seeking information and contacts in global health. This can now be considered a very useful starting point as a reference to up-to-date and key information on many aspects of global health.

King K. Holmes, MD, PhD
William H. Foege Chair, Department of Global Health
Director, Center for AIDS and STD
Professor of Medicine and Global Health
University of Washington
Head, Infectious Diseases
Harborview Medical Center

December 2007

CARING FOR THE WORLD:
A GUIDEBOOK TO GLOBAL HEALTH OPPORTUNITIES

1 An Introduction to Global Health

We have a unique opportunity to provide services to poor, oppressed, and underserved people around the world. Today, with global travel being so common and accessible, it is easier than ever to volunteer or work internationally.

People have various motivations for seeking a global health or medical opportunity, ranging from the desire to serve less fortunate people around the world to seeking a sense of international adventure and personal discovery. A global health experience can be as short as a week or two, but some people will choose to spend a lifetime tending to the health needs of people in less developed countries. There are non-governmental organizations, religious groups, governmental agencies, and many others that can offer global health work. Furthermore, opportunities exist for undergraduate and professional students, early and mid-career professionals, as well as retired persons. Therefore, while anyone can become engaged in suitable global health activities, making the decision to embark on a global health experience and how much time to invest should be made with some background knowledge and a certain degree of motivation.

A global health experience can tax a person to her limits, both physically and emotionally, yet at the same time be the most rewarding experience of one's life. However, working overseas does not necessitate being isolated or away from family. In fact, most positions are located in more urban areas where there are other like-minded individuals, and there are ample opportunities for partners and children to participate in international experiences. Oftentimes, spouses and partners can assist with language skills, construction projects, and administrative issues, as well as provide many other possible contributions. Just lending a helping hand with a caring attitude is almost always appreciated and, hopefully, will provide an invaluable experience and a desire to return with more knowledge and skills.

With the current HIV/AIDS epidemic, many people equate global health work with addressing HIV prevention and treatment. HIV/AIDS can be a large part of a global health opportunity, particularly in Africa, Eastern Europe, or parts of Southeast Asia, but there are ample and diverse opportunities that go beyond HIV/AIDS. Programs associated with public health may range from providing clean drinking water to accessing immunization programs to delivering health education. More medically focused interventions can come from very diverse medical specialties that include surgery, obstetrics, pediatrics, emergency medicine, and family medicine. Currently, several major global health efforts are related to infectious diseases, particularly diarrheal infections, vaccine-preventable diseases, HIV, malaria, and tuberculosis. In addition, many developing countries are experiencing a growing burden of chronic, non-infectious diseases, and now suffer from both communicable and non-communicable diseases. Nonetheless, one does not need to have special training in infectious disease to have a positive and effective global health experience. A strong motivation and some good resource books will be the basis for anyone to learn and work in a global health setting.

In the remainder of this chapter, we present a brief overview of many current topics in global health. This is, however, a limited description of the many broad realms of global health and medicine. Each section is meant to be an introduction to a global health topic, since each topic could be an entire chapter or even a separate book.

A Brief History of Global Health

While the field of global health has seen an explosion of interest and funding over the past several years, Western physicians and scientists have been conducting medical and health work in tropical countries for well over a hundred years. Throughout the nineteenth century, many physicians from the United Kingdom and other colonizing countries were travelling to remote areas of the world to study diseases and treat fellow military and administrative colonialists. Dr Patrick Manson was an early British physician pioneer who left England in 1866 and studied tropical diseases in Asia for several decades. By the end of the nineteenth century, his research, in collaboration with Ronald Ross in India, established the female mosquito as the transmitter of the malaria-causing organism, *Plasmodia*. The English physician Patrick Manson was instrumental in promoting the study of global health and medicine. He then founded the London School of Tropical Medicine in 1898, and, after his death, came to be considered the founder of tropical medicine.[1]

In 1874 the fourth International Sanitary Conference in Vienna proposed an idea for a permanent International Commission on Epidemics. In 1902 an International Sanitary Bureau in Washington was formed, and the Bureau became the precursor of the Pan American Health Organization. A year later the first international public health office, called the L'Office International d'Hygiène Publique (OIHP – the 'Paris Office'), was formed at a conference. The Paris Office opened in 1909, and it joined the need for controlling infectious diseases with securing public health improvements. In 1920 a separate health office was formed under the auspices of the League of Nations to provide technical support to help solve national health problems. It was called the League of Nations Health Office (LNHO).

In 1948, just after the end of the Second World War, global health received a major boost through the founding of the World Health Organization (WHO) as a specialized agency of the United Nations. The WHO was formed by combining the Pan American Health Organization, the Paris Office, and the LNHO. The WHO's mission was and still is 'the attainment by all peoples of the highest possible level of health.' The WHO served as the coordinating agency to monitor outbreaks of infections and combat diseases by distributing vaccines. The WHO played a leading role in the fight against smallpox, and certified global smallpox eradication in May 1980.[2] Since then the WHO has continued to be the primary multinational agency focusing on global health issues.

In 1978 the WHO and United Nations Children's Fund (UNICEF) held an historic conference in Alma Ata, in Kazakhstan (in the former Soviet Union).[3] The conference described primary health care as a new approach to health and medicine that should be made universally accessible to all individuals and families. One of the key components of the primary health care model was equitable distribution, and the attendees at Alma Ata declared that basic medical services should be available to all people irrespective of their ability to pay. At the conclusion of this conference, there was enthusiasm to provide basic health services to all people, particularly those in developing countries. However, there was still financial reluctance to invest in global health programs.

Another breakthrough came in 1993 with the publication of the World

Bank's annual World Development Report, entitled *Investing in Health*.[4] The report outlined the economic benefits of investing in health as a method of improving economic development and growth in developing countries. With the World Bank's approval, national governments of developing countries received the financial justification to invest in their health sectors. However, many of these countries already mired in national debt from World Bank and International Monetary Fund (IMF) loans, and they had few resources to invest in health care infrastructure.[5]

At the end of the twentieth century, with the global HIV/AIDS epidemic drawing much attention, the interest and funding for global health began to rapidly expand.[6] At the forefront of these efforts has been the Bill and Melinda Gates Foundation, which pledged $8.5 billion dollars for global health and medicine from 1999 to 2007,[7] roughly equivalent to the budget of the WHO over the same period. More recently, the U.S. President's Emergency Plan for AIDS Relief (PEPFAR) from the George W. Bush administration has pledged $15 billion over 5 years to help select, primarily African, countries to fight the HIV/AIDS epidemic. Many other foundations, non-profit organizations, and governmental organizations have been instrumental in promoting and funding global health initiatives and programs.*

Global health has become so popular over the past several years that prominent politicians, including Jimmy Carter, Tony Blair, and Bill Clinton, as well as celebrities, including Bono and Richard Gere, have been championing the push for more global health efforts. Never before has there been such a radical shift in funding and attention in health care and medicine as there has been towards the evolving field of global health and medicine. Yet, at the same time, there is a widening gap in medical care between more-developed and less-developed countries, and the rich and poor within some countries.

World Health Organization and Other Global Health Organizations

The World Health Organization (WHO) is a body of the United Nations and considered the world's flagship organization for global health and medicine. The WHO is comprised of 193 member countries and is headquartered in Geneva, Switzerland. There are also six regional

---

*All dollar amounts in U.S. currency, unless stated otherwise.

offices (Europe, Eastern Mediterranean, Africa, Southeast Asia, Western Pacific, and the Americas) around the world.

WHO policy is determined at the World Health Assembly, which is held annually in May. The Director-General and the Secretariat prepare reports on current health topics to be discussed at the World Health Assembly. There is also an Executive Board, comprised of 32 technical experts, who are voted upon to serve a 3-year term, to determine the direction and actions of the WHO. The current Director-General is Margaret Chan from China.

The WHO contributes to global health and medicine through two major methods. The first is by providing technical help, such as epidemiological surveillance, international standardization of drugs and vaccines, and dissemination of health knowledge. The second is by means of assistance through specific services to governments at the request of member countries. These services could be programs, such as developing coordination of regional training, or holding meetings, such as bringing specific health experts together from a world region.

Other prominent global health organizations include the following:

1 Other United Nations agencies include UNICEF, United Nations High Commission for Refugees (UNHCR), United Nations Development Program (UNDP), World Food Program (WFP), United Nations Environment Program (UNEP), United Nations Population Fund (UNFPA), and the United Nations Centre for Human Settlements (Habitat).
2 The World Bank and its Human Development Network work on health and development projects. The Network includes regional offices and often involves regional development banks.
3 Multilateral quasi-governmental agencies include the Global Fund for AIDS, Tuberculosis, and Malaria (GFATM) and the Global Alliance for Vaccines and Immunizations (GAVI).
4 National development agencies and government initiatives, such as the United States Agency for International Development (USAID) and the Canadian International Development Agency (CIDA), provide both bilateral and multilateral aid and assistance. Similarly, some government initiatives such as the United States Peace Corps and the recent PEPFAR program promote and address various health issues.
5 Non-governmental organizations (NGOs) include private volunteer organizations (PVOs) and religiously affiliated organizations, such as

CARE, Oxfam, PATH, and Médecins sans Frontières (Doctors without Borders).

6 Foundations, such as the Bill and Melinda Gates Foundation, Aga Khan Foundation, Rockefeller Foundation, Kellogg Foundation, Ford Foundation, and the Wellcome Trust, often serve as financiers of global health efforts.

Millennium Development Goals

The Millennium Development Goals (MDGs) are a set of values and principles that reaffirm the common bonds of humankind. In September 2000, at the United Nations Millennium Summit, world leaders from 189 countries agreed to a set of eight time-bound and measurable goals for addressing issues of poverty, illness, poor education, malnutrition, women's rights, and environmental degradation. They also focused on improving human rights, good governance, and democracy. The Millennium Development Goals were then adopted as a set of guiding principles of the United Nations Organization.[8]

The eight MDGs and their 18 quantifiable targets are as follows:

Goal 1: Eradicate extreme poverty and hunger
- Reduce by half (between 1990 to 2015) the proportion of people living on less than a dollar a day.
- Reduce by half (between 1990 to 2015) the proportion of people who suffer from hunger.

Goal 2: Achieve universal primary education
- Ensure that all boys and girls complete a full course of primary schooling.

Goal 3: Promote gender equality and empower women
- Eliminate gender disparity in primary and secondary education preferably by 2005, and at all levels by 2015.

Goal 4: Reduce child mortality
- Reduce by two-thirds the mortality rate among children under 5 years of age by 2015.

Goal 5: Improve maternal health
- Reduce by three-quarters the maternal mortality ratio by 2015.

Goal 6: Combat HIV/AIDS, malaria, and other diseases
- Halt and begin to reverse the spread of HIV/AIDS.
- Halt and begin to reverse the incidence of malaria and other major diseases.

Goal 7: Ensure environmental sustainability
- Integrate the principles of sustainable development into country policies and programs; reverse loss of environmental resources.
- Reduce by half (between 1990 to 2015) the proportion of people without sustainable access to safe drinking water.
- Achieve significant improvement in lives of at least 100 million slum dwellers, by 2020.

Goal 8: Develop a Global Partnership for Development
- Develop further an open, rule-based, predictable, non-discriminatory trading and financial system. This includes a commitment to good governance, development, and poverty reduction – both nationally and internationally.
- Address the special needs of the least developed countries. This includes tariff- and quota-free access for least developed countries' exports; an enhanced program of debt relief for highly indebted countries and cancellation of official bilateral debt; and more generous official development assistance for countries committed to reducing poverty.
- Address the special needs of landlocked countries and small island developing states.
- Deal comprehensively with the debt problems of developing countries through national and international measures in order to make debt sustainable in the long term.
- In cooperation with developing countries, develop and implement strategies for decent and productive work for youth.
- In cooperation with pharmaceutical companies, provide access to affordable essential drugs in developing countries.
- In cooperation with the private sector, make available the benefits of new technologies, especially information and communications.

Recent reports show that some of these achievements have been reached, while others still have a long way to go.[9] One of the vast improvements is a reduction in extreme poverty from 31.6% in 1990 to 19.2% in 2004.[9] However, when analysing these figures by region, there are significant concerns that improvements in sub-Saharan Africa are occurring too slowly. Other positive progress has been made in increasing the number of children attending primary school and in reducing child mortality.

Unfortunately, there are areas where little improvement has occurred. For example, 500,000 women still die every year from childbirth, increasing numbers of people are dying from HIV/AIDS, income inequality has continued to rise, and there are growing concerns over global climate change and its potential effects on the ecosystem.

The Millennium Development Goals provide a benchmark for improving economic and social development, but unfortunately, many goals will not be attained without significant global commitment and partnership in attaining them. The measures that will be achieved will depend on political will and the determination of people to improve the conditions of the poorest in the world.

HIV/AIDS

The current HIV/AIDS pandemic presents the greatest human health disaster of our time. Over 25 million people have already died from HIV/AIDS.[10] At the end of 2005 nearly 35 million people worldwide were living with HIV, and 15 million children have lost at least one parent to HIV/AIDS. The global adult HIV seroprevalence rate had reached 1%, indicating that 1 of every 100 adults carries HIV, and this rate has continued to climb (Figure 1.1); during 2005 another 4.1 million people became newly infected with HIV, and an estimated 2.8 million HIV-infected persons died.[10,11] Although lives are being extended by antiretroviral medications, the pandemic has continued to grow. In some southern African countries, HIV has been estimated to infect almost one-third of adults.

The global fight against HIV/AIDS turned a corner after entering the new millennium. In 2001 leaders from 189 member states of the U.N. General Assembly adopted the Declaration of Commitment on HIV/AIDS. The Declaration identified specific targets for effective HIV prevention, care, and support needed to reverse the global epidemic by 2015.[10] Access to antiretroviral treatment in low- and middle-income countries increased from 240,000 people in 2001 to 1.3 million people in 2005. By 2005 the total expenditure among low- and middle-income countries for HIV/AIDS had reached $8.3 billion per year.

The Global Fund to Fight AIDS, Tuberculosis, and Malaria was created in December 2002 as a partnership between governments, civil society, the private sector, and affected communities. By 2006 the Global Fund had approved a total of 350 grants for HIV programs to government and civil society partners in 128 countries.[10] In 2005 the Global Fund had disbursed an estimated $1.1 billion for HIV/AIDS. Additionally, the World Bank had provided a cumulative total of more than $2.5 billion to HIV programs.

Figure 1.1: Estimated number of adults and children living with HIV, by region, 1990–2007

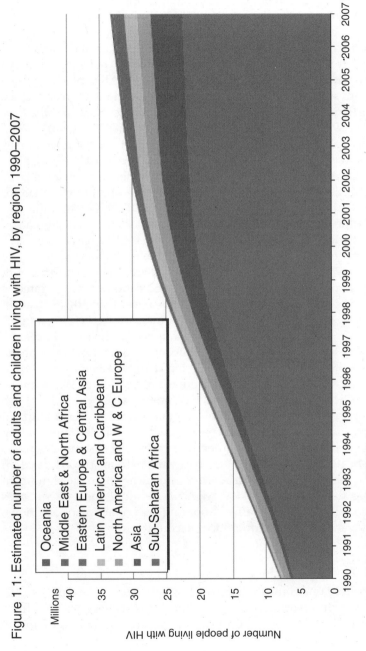

Legend:
- Oceania
- Middle East & North Africa
- Eastern Europe & Central Asia
- Latin America and Caribbean
- North America and W & C Europe
- Asia
- Sub-Saharan Africa

Millions

Number of people living with HIV

Reproduced by kind permission of UNAIDS.

In 2003 the U.S. President's Emergency Plan for AIDS Relief pledged $15 billion dollars over five years.[13] The U.S. contributions to global HIV/AIDS increased from $840 million in fiscal year 2001 to over $3 billion in fiscal year 2006. Most importantly, the government agreed to fund antiretroviral medications for HIV-infected persons requiring treatment, who had been left out of previous HIV/AIDS plans. By 2006 the program was providing antiretroviral medications to over 500,000 people in 15 of the most affected countries in Africa, Asia, and the Caribbean. The PEPFAR program is, however, not without controversy. Despite the plan's reluctance to provide support for commercial sex workers and the requirement to purchase higher cost U.S. drugs, the program has proved extremely valuable in the global fight against HIV/AIDS. In his 2008 State of the Union Address, President Bush called for another $30 billion over the next 5 years for the PEPFAR program.

Despite the progress, there is still a long way to go. At the end of 2005, among low- and middle-income countries, HIV medications had reached only one in five people who needed them.[10] Despite increasing access to HIV medication in sub-Saharan Africa, most countries with high HIV seroprevalence rates had HIV medication coverage rates of less than 25%, and many had coverage rates of less than 10%.[10] In addition, only 9% of HIV-positive pregnant women were receiving antiretroviral prophylaxis to prevent HIV transmission to their newborns. As a result, 26% of infants born to HIV-infected mothers in some of the most affected countries were born infected with HIV. Finally, the financial resource requirements for 2007 were estimated to be $18.1 billion – this is $8 billion more than the projected resources.

The way forward will be multifaceted and complex. Major shifts in addressing global health and HIV issues, which include (1) providing free HIV medications, (2) strengthening health care systems, (3) training more health care providers, (4) addressing extreme poverty, and (5) expanding basic science research, will be necessary to make significant and lasting reductions in the HIV/AIDS pandemic.[13] The consequences of inaction will inequitably affect poor and marginalized populations, particularly in low- and middle-income countries.

Tuberculosis

Approximately one-third of all people have a latent tuberculosis (TB) infection, which can reactivate at any time. Roughly 95% of individuals with active TB, and nearly all of the deaths due to TB, occur in the developing world.[14] The incidence of TB is highest in sub-Saharan African countries with high HIV seroprevalence rates, since HIV can reactivate latent TB. Tuberculosis kills more than one and a half million people each year.[15]

Tuberculosis has been recognized as a human health problem for centuries, and several methods of treating TB have been tried. In the 1950s and 1960s the first anti-TB medications were introduced, and they were very effective at treating TB, especially since there were few antibiotic-resistant strains of TB in circulation. Since the 1960s, when TB became less menacing in the developed countries, little attention has been given to improving or developing new anti-TB therapies. After decades of neglect among the more resource-limited countries, by the late 1980s, it had become obvious that a TB epidemic was occurring.[16]

In 1994 the WHO launched DOTS (Directly Observed Therapy, Short-course) as a public health–based management strategy aimed at controlling TB. Since TB is a very slow-growing organism, several months of antibiotic therapy are needed to treat an infection. DOTS focuses on identification of the most infectious (smear positive) patients and helped ensure that patients took their full course of medication. Although the program has some shortcomings, most experts agree that DOTS has been successful in most settings with patients who do not have multidrug-resistant TB (MDR-TB) and who are not HIV co-infected. Under these typical settings, targeting TB-infected patients with DOTS can reduce the annual TB occurrence by 6% to 10%.[14]

The WHO recommends a 6-month course of anti-TB therapy, as specified by the DOTS protocol, but this may result in incomplete treatment for some patients and in significant burdens on struggling health care systems for some countries. Despite the limitations, many specialists concur that DOTS is the most feasible treatment program available in resource-poor settings.

As HIV has spread throughout Africa and Asia, TB rates are dramatically increasing in those regions.[17] In some countries, TB has become the chief cause of death among individuals infected with HIV. Those public health systems are being double taxed by soaring numbers of TB-infected individuals and already high rates of HIV. This intersection of TB and HIV has become a new global challenge, and particularly so in Africa and Asia. Unfortunately, DOTS has not evolved to address HIV and TB dual-infected people.[16]

As patients cease taking any or all of their TB medications as their health improves, drug-resistant strains of TB become more apparent.

There have been warnings about the global problem of multiple drug-resistant strains of TB (MDR-TB). Reports of an outbreak of extremely drug-resistant TB (XDR-TB) among mostly HIV-positive individuals in South Africa have raised major concerns about the new, deadly strain that could spread throughout the African continent and beyond.[18] Few people in developing countries have second-line treatment for MDR-TB or XDR-TB available to them.

Recent alliances and collaborative efforts among organizations active in TB control, research, and development are seeking to improve treatments. These organizations, led by the Global Fund for AIDS, Tuberculosis, and Malaria, have created unprecedented monetary resources to develop TB control strategies in resource-poor areas and to finance the development of new medications for treating TB. Controlling the expanding drug-resistant TB epidemic may depend on developing new approaches and discovering new TB therapies.[19]

Malaria

Malaria causes more than 300 million acute illnesses and at least 1 million deaths annually. Most malaria-endemic countries lie along the equator, and the hardest hit are the tropical countries in Africa.[20] Malaria, along with HIV/AIDS and tuberculosis, has become one of the primary public health challenges in developing equatorial countries.

Among the millions of adults that become infected each year, malaria usually causes significant morbidity. Most malaria-related fatalities occur in children. Those children who do survive an episode of severe cerebral malaria are at risk for permanent brain damage, seizure disorders, and other neurological sequelae.[21]

Malaria is both preventable and treatable. Several evidence-based, cost-effective interventions can significantly reduce the incidence of malaria. When these interventions are used aggressively in malaria-endemic areas, they can have a notable bearing on the morbidity and mortality caused by malaria.

Malaria is caused by a parasite that is transmitted by female mosquitoes. The mosquitoes primarily bite people at dawn and dusk. The proper use and maintenance of mosquito bed nets provides a physical barrier to protect people against infected mosquitoes. When treated with an insecticide, such as permethrin, these bed nets become significantly more effective at preventing malaria infections. Furthermore, the cost of such a simple and effective intervention is less than $3 per bed net.

Indoor spraying of an insecticide, such as DDT, is another effective method of reducing malaria cases. The insecticide kills all mosquitoes and therefore reduces malaria transmission by controlling the vector. However, because of concerns about the DDT compound, this approach has not been without controversy. Yet, reliable data confirm the efficacy and safety of indoor residual spraying with insecticide to control malaria when properly implemented.[30]

For the past half-century, chloroquine has been the most accessible anti-malarial drug available. At the end of the 1950s, however, resistance to chloroquine started to emerge among the deadliest strain of the malaria parasite, *Plasmodium falciparum*.[23] Today, chloroquine is still used in much of Asia, South America, and the Horn of Africa for the treatment of *Plasmodium vivax* malaria, but not for *P. falciparum* malaria.

In 2005 artemisinin-based combination treatments (ACTs) became the first line of therapy for *P. falciparum* malaria in many malaria-endemic countries. The ACTs work effectively and rapidly, and they have fewer adverse effects. Unfortunately, they are more expensive than the single-agent therapies, and accessibility of the effective medication has been a major challenge.[23]

A delay in the administration of effective anti-malarial treatment causes the majority of deaths from severe malaria. When a young child becomes infected with the malaria parasite, deterioration may be rapid, and without effective treatment death can occur in a matter of days or even hours. Therefore, there is a critical need to ensure that health care facilities have sufficient stocks of anti-malarial medications and supplies, and that health care personnel are trained and supervised in the rapid identification and clinical care of children with malaria. Without confidence in the health care system, parents of an infected child in rural Africa may not justify the expense of taking their child to a local health care facility to receive appropriate treatment.

Maternal and Child Health

Over 10 million children and 500,000 pregnant women die each year. Approximately 90% of childhood deaths worldwide occur in 42 developing countries, and over half of childhood deaths worldwide occur in six countries (India, Nigeria, China, Pakistan, Democratic Republic of the Congo, and Ethiopia).[24] Childhood deaths have been narrowed down to six major causes: acute respiratory infections (pneumonia), malaria, measles, gastroenteritis, perinatal death (usually sepsis), and

HIV/AIDS, with malnutrition contributing an overarching burden to all six.[24] Countries with the most maternal deaths include India, Pakistan, Ethiopia, Nigeria, Indonesia, Democratic Republic of the Congo, and Bangladesh.[25] The major causes of maternal death are severe bleeding/hemorrhage, bacterial infection and sepsis, eclampsia, and complications of abortions.[25] Two of the eight aims of the Millennium Development Goals are to 'reduce child mortality' and 'improve maternal health.'[26]

Jones et al. showed that 63% of all childhood deaths can be prevented by using technology and interventions that already exist.[27] Childhood deaths can be greatly reduced by decreasing several risk factors, such as unhygienic and unsafe environments, poor birth spacing, and lack of breastfeeding. In the mid-1990s the Integrated Management of Childhood Illnesses (IMCI) was established to promote these measures. They set guidelines to tackle several major causes of childhood deaths, such as malaria, pneumonia, and gastroenteritis. They also combined the diagnostic and treatment aspects of these illnesses with nutrition, immunizations, and other influences on child health.

Maternal and reproductive health continues to be a highly neglected issue in many developing countries. Over 99% of maternal deaths occur in developing countries, and approximately 50 million women suffer from acute pregnancy-related complications. Particularly striking is that over 56 million unwanted pregnancies occur every year, leading to 42 million abortions and 74,000 deaths annually in mothers and 4 million neonatal deaths and 3 million stillborn deaths.[28,29] The Safe Mother Initiative, started in 1987, concentrated on addressing the issues of maternal mortality in developing countries. A new initiative, called the Integrated Management of Pregnancy and Childbirth (IMPAC), was launched to address the issues around neonatal and maternal mortality by strengthening care during childbirth, including having a skilled birth attendant available, and by instituting care for both the mother and child after delivery.

Mental Health

Neuropsychiatric conditions, which include psychiatric, neurological, and behavioural disorders, affect hundreds of millions of people worldwide and account for 1.2 million deaths per year.[30] Depression and other common mental disorders cause significant personal impairment due to their chronic disabling nature. Together, they are responsible for an estimated 14% of the global burden of disease.[31] After communicable diseases, neuropsychiatric conditions cause the highest global burden of disease and contribute more to global morbidity than either cardiovascular disease or cancer. Not counted in these statistics are the 800,000 people who commit suicide each year.

In 2005 the WHO reported on the inadequate availability of mental health services worldwide.[24] Their finding was particularly apparent for low- and middle-income countries, which contain 85% of the world's population. For example, there were approximately 89,000 psychiatrists for 879 million people in the European Region, but only 1,800 psychiatrists for 702 million African people. In addition, the average number of psychiatric hospital beds was 13-fold greater among high-income countries compared with low-income countries. Among low-income countries, over 95% of people were living in a country with less than one psychiatrist and one psychologist per 100,000 people.

Most low- and middle-income countries have allocated very scarce financial, personnel, and infrastructure resources for mental health care.[32] In addition, almost one-third of countries had no mental health legislation, and 20% did not have policies or programs to guide their services. Incorporating mental health care services into the primary health care system is important for several reasons. Mental disorders are independently associated with higher all-cause mortality risk and with risk factors for acquiring communicable diseases; in addition, mental disorders contribute to accidental and non-accidental injuries.[24] Therefore, treating mental disorders would not only reduce the global burden of neuropsychiatric conditions, but doing so would also help reduce the morbidity and mortality of other diseases. Recent analyses have suggested that treating mental health problems would be cost-effective in developing countries, and could be done with an additional $2 to $4 per person per year.[33]

After recognizing the extent of this neglected problem, the efforts to reduce the global burden of mental health problems and incorporate these services into standard primary care have increased. The WHO launched the mental health Global Action Programme (mhGAP) to focus on enhancing countries' capacity to combat stigma, reducing the burden of mental disorders, and promoting mental health.[34] Efforts are now under way to better understand the interactions between mental health and other conditions, as well as developing appropriate mental health interventions. One proposal recommends conducting research to assess interventions that can be delivered by people who are not mental health professionals.[25] Ameliorating the large global mental health burden can be successfully achieved, but it will take a long-term commitment from the global health community, funding agencies, and national governments.

Primary Health Care (PHC)

A health system based on PHC cannot, and I repeat, cannot be realized, cannot be developed, cannot function and simply cannot exist without a network of hospitals with responsibilities for supporting PHC; promoting community health development action and continuing education of all categories of health personnel; and research.

– Halfdan Mahler, Former Director-General, World Health Organization

The concept of primary health care was launched at the Alma Ata Conference in 1978 with the slogan 'Health for All by the Year 2000.'[35] The participants of the conference proposed providing better access to inexpensive and simple health care services to improve the health of all people. The basic concept is that primary health care should be the first level of contact with a national health system, and the quality of the services should be based on the economic development of each individual country.[36] Health care workers would gain the necessary primary health care knowledge, skills, and attitudes to help their communities achieve specific health goals, which would be based on economic resources.

The Alma Ata Declaration[35] states: Primary Health Care is essential health care based on practical, scientifically sound and socially acceptable methods and technology, made universally accessible to individuals and families in the community, through their full participation and at a cost that the community and country can afford to maintain at every state of their development, in the spirit of self-reliance and self-determination. It forms an integral part both of the country's health system, of which it is the central function and main focus, and of the overall social and economic development of the community.

There are eight essential core components to primary health care that together form the acronym 'MEDICINE.'[37]

- Maternal and child health care, including family planning, antenatal care, and clinics for children under 5 years of age.
- Education in the language that people understand.
- Drugs incorporated into a country's essential drug list.

- Immunization against vaccine-preventable diseases.
- Common disease management, such as Integrated Management of Childhood Illnesses (IMCI) and Integrated Management of Pregnancy and Childbirth (IMPAC).
- Indigenous epidemiology, disease treatment, and control.
- Nutrition support, promoting breastfeeding, safe food supplies, and micronutrient support.
- Environmental practices, including sanitation and protection of safe drinking supplies.

The key values of primary health care include several principles. First, there is a principle of equity – health services should be equally accessible to all people, whether they live in rural areas, urban slums, or in racially isolated communities. Second, the community should be involved in the decision-making process and be considered a full partner in all phases of planning, implementation, and evaluation. Third, there should be a focus on preventive services and the promotion of good health. As an example, many years ago, Chinese physicians were paid only when their patients were well and stopped receiving their salary when their patients became ill. Fourth, appropriate technology should be used if it is available, affordable, and sustainable. Fifth, there should be a multisectoral approach to health that includes cooperation with other local, regional, and national government agencies, such as education, water development, agriculture, women's affairs, and housing. To allow for an effective, comprehensive approach to improving health, it is paramount that open communication with all other involved parties occurs. Sixth, decentralization of decision-making is required to allow for appropriate interventions and priorities to be made by local groups, and for their actions to be tailored to their local situation and needs. Finally, leadership is required to promote health and to bring this concept of decentralized decision-making into the mainstream of medical and health education. The health professional can initiate change, and involve and mobilize others to create networks required to develop effective community leadership in health.

Obviously, providing 'Health for All by the Year 2000' was not achieved. Although there are many complicated reasons why this was not achieved, Hall and Taylor highlight four major reasons: (1) PHC was felt to be a cheap and inadequate form of health care; (2) civil war, natural disasters, and HIV/AIDS made it impossible to maintain appropriate PHC systems; (3) the political will was lacking; and (4) donor governments were reluctant to fund broad-based programs.[38] The need for creating a primary care infrastructure in developing countries has never abated, and with recent increases in funding and interest these initiatives may have a greater chance at future successes.

Poverty, Politics, and Global Health

The strong association between poverty and poor health has long been recognized. In 1980 Samuel Preston noted that countries with average annual incomes rising to about $1,000 per capita had associated increases in life expectancy.[39] However, above this average annual income, few additional years of life were gained with increases in wealth. Lant Pritchett and Larry Summers, in their classical paper entitled 'Wealthier Is Healthier,' observed that 40% of cross-country differences in mortality can be explained by the growth in average annual income.[40] They estimated that a 1% increase in worldwide income would lead to a global reduction of 33,000 infant and 55,000 child deaths annually.

Over the past decade, there has been increasing evidence that better health leads to greater development and wealth. The strong evidence culminated in the published work by the Macroeconomic Commission on Health, led by Dr Jeffery Sachs. As suggested by David Bloom and David Canning, four key mechanisms can explain the health to wealth mechanism: (1) increased productivity gains from having better health, (2) increased investment in education and human capital, (3) increased investment in physical capital, and (4) benefits from the demographic dividend as a larger population moves through the labour-force ages.[41]

Politics also play a significant role in medicine and health. Health care is one of the largest expenditures for governments, and the United States spends approximately 15% of its gross domestic product (GDP) on health. The choice of a country's financing model for health care often defines its social care and support network. Similarly, greater social and economic inequality, racism, and regionalism may lead to poorer health conditions and outcomes.

Politics could also have a significant impact on changing priorities and reducing preventable deaths. When one considers that the U.S.-led war in Iraq costs approximately $5.8 billion per month, it becomes a matter of priorities whether or not we can significantly lessen the scourge of human suffering and death through global health efforts.[42] The relationship between poor health and human suffering can also be circular. In the movie *An Inconvenient Truth*, by former U.S. Vice-

President Al Gore, links are drawn between climate change and famine, then between famine and poverty, and then between poverty and war.

Thus, poverty, politics, and global health are intertwined and interlinked. The ability to consider the broader determinants of health is essential in achieving an optimal state of global health.

Social Determinants of Health

People who are poor live fewer years and have more illness than those who are rich. This inherent inequity has given rise to a new field whose aim is to examine the social determinants of health. Donkin et al. showed that men and women in more affluent working classes have almost half the risk of serious illness and premature death compared with their poorer counterparts.[43] The effects of poverty, which start with nutrition and education for a child, continue through adulthood with poorer working and living conditions, and less support for retirement. The effects of poverty are cumulative with time.

Stress not only can impair one's health, but also lead to premature death. Poor childhood nutrition, even during fetal development, may lead to poor cardiovascular outcomes in adulthood – a theory known as the Barker hypothesis.[44] Likewise, early and healthy childhood development can have a significant positive impact on brain growth, long-term social development, educational ability, and productivity. Therefore, ensuring adequate growth and potential development requires specific attention to children.

Racism, discrimination, stigmatization, and unemployment can lead to issues and failures of people to participate in activities such as job training, education, civic duty, and successfully navigating social services.[45] Mentally ill children who are left in group homes and jailed prisoners are particularly vulnerable to social exclusion. Coupled with poverty, these stigmas lead to increased rates of divorce, disability, mental and physical illness, and drug and alcohol addiction.[46]

Finally, social networks are seen as an important contributor to good health. These networks help provide strong emotional support, which has a protective effect on health. Furthermore, when people in communities trust each other – a concept known as social cohesion – these elements lead to decreased levels of violence and expansion of community development programs, which in turn improve health.[47]

The social determinants of health have gained increased attention and risen in importance in global health, which has led to the creation of a new division by that name of the World Health Organization. The WHO division released *Social Determinants of Health: The Solid Facts* (2nd ed.), edited by Richard Wilkinson and Michael Marmot, which highlights some of these determinants and roles of social structure, and describes the root causes or poor health.[48] Social structures and the factors that underlie social structures are important aspects in determining good individual health outcomes.

Ethnocultural Determinants of Health

One of the joys of global health is the exposure to different cultures, ethnicities, and beliefs. This means understanding how different cultures understand health issues and implement programs. There is an increasing recognition, even among domestic populations, that health professionals need to be sensitive to the needs of different population groups. It is important to recognize that certain populations may have higher risks of particular diseases, such as sickle cell disease in people who live in endemic malaria regions or cystic fibrosis in northern European descendants.

It is also important to recognize that health care and health systems may be viewed differently. For example, people in many cultures do not visits physicians first for a health problem, but instead consult a traditional healer. Other practices may seem cruel, such as female genital mutilation in northern Nigeria or coin rubbing in China and Vietnam to scare away evil spirits, but their support may be quite common within those countries.

Some people may have different religious or spiritual beliefs, and as a result may see Western medicine as a 'bizarre practice.' For example, many Chinese people believe in Taoism, where good health is achieved by balancing two dynamically opposing forces: the 'yin' and the 'yang.' Thus, when a child has a 'fever' and 'chills,' they believe a child is cold and they bundle the child to keep him warm.

In many places, traditional medications are derived from herbs, tree roots, and other natural objects. Many of these 'herbal remedies' have found their way into modern medicine. Taxol is a drug currently used in the treatment of lung, ovarian, breast, head, and neck cancers that comes from the bark of the Pacific yew tree, *Taxus brevifolia*. The newest generation of anti-malarial drugs is artemisinin, which is derived from leaves of the sweet wormwood tree, *Artemisia annua*.

Along with traditions and medications, it is also important to recognize the role of cultural practices in delivering health care. For example, a male physician should never see the hair of a Muslim woman, and an elderly male is considered to be the principal decision-maker in many cultures. The recognition of these roles is important in gaining acceptance within communities and being effective in global health work.

Understanding a culture and community is important, but being able to communicate with the local community is paramount. Oftentimes a translator is needed to minimize confusion and gain understanding of a community's perspective on a specific problem. Interpretation of body language should be minimized in order to avoid unnecessary confusion. For example, a head nod can mean something quite different from one culture to the next. Learning basic phrases and improving one's ability to communicate in the local language dramatically opens the doors for acceptance into a community.

Finally, death is also something that has different interpretations in different societies. For example, allowing a child to die may be quite unacceptable in Western cultures, but many other cultures are less tolerable of seeing a child suffer.

Ethnocultural determinants of health do play a substantial and significant role in health care delivery and outcomes. Being sensitive and aware of these differences will help in increasing acceptance and communication in any global health endeavour.

Population, Demography, and Health

Demography is Destiny.
– Auguste Compte, seventeenth-century mathematician

In the 1790s Thomas Malthus wrote: 'it [population growth] appears ... to be decisive against the possible existence of a society, all the members of which should live in ease, happiness, and comparative leisure, and feel no anxiety about providing the means of subsistence for themselves and families.'[49] Malthus and those that followed him, such as Paul Ehrlich, were pessimists who believed that population growth would lead to overuse of resources and then to mass starvation. Some of the current neo-Malthusians believe that climate change is a result of gross overuse of resources.

Contrary to Malthus, there are those who may be called the population optimists and who believe that technology will consistently outpace population size. As the population grows, ingenuity will also

Figure 1.2: The demographic transition

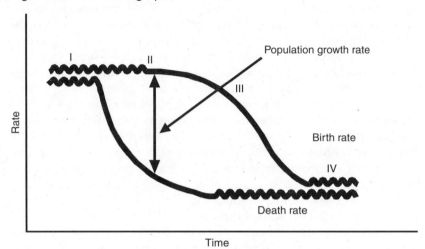

increase, and the economies of scale will allow for new technology to meet the ever-changing needs of the population. They generally believe that there's a technological solution that can relieve any resource constraint.

Population growth became more rapid after the industrial revolution in the second half of the nineteenth century. Ten thousand years ago, in 8,000 BC, the global population growth rate was approximately eight people per year. In 1750 the global population growth rate had risen to about 81,000 people per year. In 1927 the global population was expanding by about 8 million people per year. In 2000 the global population was growing by 83 million people per year. Currently, the U.N. Population Prospects project the global population to grow to 9.1 billion people by 2050.[50]

The significant growth of the global population has been facilitated by the demographic transition. During rapid population growth a country goes through a four-stage transformation (see Figure 1.2). In stage I, a country will have both a high birth rate and death rate. In stage II, the death rate begins to decline, often from improvements in child health, while the birth rate remains high. In stage III, a country's birth rate begins to fall and becomes more in line with the country's low death rate. And finally, in stage IV, both the birth rate and death rate remain at low levels. During stages II and III, a rapid rise in the population level occurs.

Countries that undergo a demographic transition have a population that lives longer. This, in turn, has led to a transition in epidemiological trends and major causes of morbidity and mortality within a population. For example, countries that have undergone a demographic transition tend to place less emphasis on childhood infectious diseases and 'diseases of the poor.' Instead, they tend to focus on the chronic diseases of the more affluent, such as cancer, diabetes, and cardiovascular disease. An aging population implies a growing need to find methods to care for the elderly, and an increasing burden of caring for the elderly being placed upon the 'working-age' population. These demographic influences will cause greater difficulties in providing and improving services for the elderly, and will remain one of the most important global health and development challenges of this century.

Human Rights

> Whereas recognition of the inherent dignity of the equal and inalienable rights of all members of the human family is the foundation of freedom, justice and peace in the world.
>
> Whereas disregard and contempt for human rights have resulted in barbarous acts which have outraged the conscience of mankind, and the advent of a world in which human beings shall enjoy freedom of speech and belief, and freedom from fear and want has been proclaimed as the highest aspiration of the common people.
>
> – Preamble to the Universal Declaration of Human Rights,
> U.N. General Assembly, 1948

At the heart of modern human rights lies a broader, societal approach to the complex problem of human well-being. The question that the human rights movement has brought forth is the following: What are the societal and government roles and responsibilities to promote human welfare? Answers to this question lead to two main approaches, which are embodied in the following two branches of the Universal Declaration of Human Rights: (1) the International Covenant on Civil and Political Rights (ICCPR) and (2) the International Covenant on Economic, Social and Cultural Rights (ICESCR). The ICCPR has focused on the issue of what governments should not do. By way of example, governments should not torture, discriminate, invade privacy, imprison inhumanely, ban information, stop people from gathering, etc. In contrast, the ICESCR has focused on a government's minimum obligation to ensure a basic standard of life, including education, housing, food, adequate labour conditions, and access to health care.

Protecting and promoting human rights is essential to maintaining health. The human rights approach to health has included several large movements, such as sexual and reproductive health rights as well as the demand for access to HIV/AIDS medications. These movements have highlighted the ability of a human rights approach to successfully tackle large and important global health issues.

Several organizations have become prominent in the struggle to maintain and ensure human rights. Some organizations, such as Human Rights Watch (www.hrw.org) and the United Nations (www.un.int), assist in exposing international human rights violations. Other organizations, such as the Nobel Peace Prize–recipient Physicians for Human Rights (www.phr.org) and the International Rescue Committee (www.theirc.org), provide national and global assistance for various human rights issues, including refugee and immigration assistance. Médecins sans Frontières (Doctors without Borders) has spearheaded the concept of access to essential medicines, as part of an individual's right to access to health.

Conflicts, Disasters, and Refugees

Health and medicine, as related to conflicts, disasters, and refugees, has always been of great need around the world. Recently, these issues have gained increasing publicity after the tsunami in southeast Asia, Hurricane Katrina, and the humanitarian crisis in the Darfur region of Sudan.

The greatest need for outside health and medical interventions lies in locations where the medical infrastructure is already being stretched beyond its capacity. In these situations, a medical provider not only has to understand the medical environment, but also know how to deal with limited resources. In these situations, many deaths are due to infectious diseases related to poor sanitary conditions and contaminated drinking water. Medical providers as well as additional medical supplies, particularly antibiotics, can be very helpful in these situations.

Predicting a natural disaster is almost impossible, but preparing for such catastrophes can be performed with regular assessments and evaluations of the health and medical systems. However, health needs assessments are often not conducted, or done with very limited financial support, and can lead to horrible consequences. To address these needs, in 1997, a group of humanitarian non-governmental organizations and the Red Cross and Red Crescent movements launched the Sphere Project to tackle how to properly address and alleviate human suffering out of calamity, and to outline how people in disaster situations should be treated both with dignity and a right to assistance.[51] The International Rescue Committee, Médecins sans Frontières (Doctors without Borders), the International Red Cross and Red Crescent Societies, the American Rescue Committee, and Médecins du Monde (Doctors of the World) are a few of the many non-governmental organizations that work on conflict, disaster, and refugee issues around the world. In addition to providing direct medical care, they also assist with addressing preventive care including immunizations and sanitation needs and establishing a clean water supply, and also providing food for hungry refugees. Unfortunately, the demand for this important work will extend long into the foreseeable future.

REFERENCES

1 Haynes DM. *Imperial Medicine: Patrick Manson and the Conquest of Tropical Diseases.* Philadelphia: University of Pennsylvania Press, 2001.

2 World Health Organization (WHO). 33rd World Health Assembly, resolution WHA33.3, 8 May 1980. www.wpro.who.int/rcm/en/archives/rc31/wpr/rc31_r79.htm

3 WHO. Alma Ata 1978: Primary Health Care, HFA Sr. No. 1. www.who.int/hpr/NPH/docs/declaration_almaata.pdf

4 World Bank. *World Development Report 1993: Investing in Health.* Oxford: Oxford University Press, 1993.

5 Peabody JW. Economic reform and health sector policy: Lessons from structural adjustment programs. *Social Science and Medicine* 1996; 43:823–835.

6 Jon Cohen. The new world of global health. *Science* 2006; 311:162–167.

7 Bill and Melinda Gates Foundation. Global Health Grants. www.gatesfoundation.org/GlobalHealth/Grants/default.htm?showYear=2008 (last accessed 25 Jan. 2008).

8 United Nations. The Millennium Development Goals and the United Nations Role. www.un.org/millenniumgoals/MDGs-FACTSHEET1.pdf (last accessed 15 Jan. 2008).

 9 United Nations. *The Millennium Development Goals Report 2007*. New York: United Nations, 2007.
10 Joint U.N. Programme on HIV/AIDS. *2006 Report on the Global AIDS Epidemic*. Geneva: UNAIDS, 2006.
11 Joint U.N. Programme on HIV/AIDS. *2007 AIDS Epidemic Update*. Geneva: UNAIDS, 2007.
12 U.S. President's Emergency Plan for AIDS Relief. Making a Difference: Supporting Antiretroviral Treatment. 2006. www.state.gov/documents/organization/67502.pdf
13 Kim JY, Farmer P. AIDS in 2006 – Moving toward one world, one hope? *New England Journal of Medicine* 2006; 355:645–647.
14 Hargreaves S, Hakokongas L. Time to cough up. *Health Exchange* Aug. 2004; 8–10.
15 WHO. *Global Tuberculosis Control*. Geneva: WHO, 2006.
16 Chaisson R, DeLuca A. Going beyond DOTS to control dual TB/HIV epidemics. *Global Aids Link* 2006; 99:6–7.
17 WHO. *Global Tuberculosis Control: Surveillance, Planning, Financing*. Geneva: WHO. 2007. WHO/HTM/TB/2007.376. www.who.int/t6/publications
18 Gandhi NR, Moll A, Sturm AW, et al. Extensively drug-resistance tuberculosis as a cause of death in patients co-infected with tuberculosis and HIV in a rural area of South Africa. *Lancet* 2006; 368:1575–1580.
19 Nardell EA, Mitnick CD. Are second-line drugs necessary to control multidrug-resistant tuberculosis? *Journal of Infectious Diseases* 2006; 194:1194–1196.
20 WHO. *World Malaria Report 2005*. Geneva: WHO, 2005.
21 WHO/Roll Back Malaria Partnership: 2001–2010 United Nations Decade to Roll Back Malaria. www.rbm.who.int
22 WHO. WHO gives indoor use of DDT a clean bill of health for controlling malaria. 15 September 2006, press release. www.who.int/mediacentre/news/releases/2006/pr50/en (last accessed 7 May 2007).
23 White N. Malaria – Time to act. *New England Journal of Medicine* 2006; 355:1956–1957.
24 Black RE, Morris SS, Bryce J. Where and why are 10 million children dying every year? *Lancet* 2003; 361:2226–2234.
25 Hill K, AbouZahr C, Wardlaw T. Estimates of maternal mortality 1995. *Bulletin of the World Health Organization* 2001; 79(3):182–193.
26 United Nations. *The Millennium Development Goals Report 2005*. New York: United Nations, 2005.
27 Jones G, Steketee RW, Black RE, Bhutta ZA, Morris SS, and the Bellagio

Child Survival Study Group. How many child deaths can we prevent this year? *Lancet* 2003; 362:65–71.

28 Daulaire N, Leidl P, Mackin L, Murphy C, Stark L. *Promises to Keep: The Toll of Unwanted Pregnancies on Women's Lives in the Developing World.* Washington, DC: Global Health Council, 2002.

29 Lawn JE, Cousens S, Zupan J. 4 million neonatal deaths: When? Where? Why? *Lancet* 2005; 365:891–900.

30 Prince M, Patel V, Saxena S, Maj M, Maselko J, Phillips MR, Rahman A. No health without mental health. *Lancet* 2007; 370:859–76.

31 WHO. *Mental Health Atlas.* Geneva: WHO, 2005.

32 Jacob KS, Sharan P, Mirza I, Garrido-Cumbrera M, Seedat S, Mari JJ, Sreenivas V, Saxena S. Mental health systems in countries: Where are we now? *Lancet* 2007; 370:1061–1077.

33 Lancet Global Mental Health Group. Scale up services for mental disorders: A call for action. Lancet 2007; 370:1241–1252.

34 WHO. Mental Health. www.who.int/mental_health/en/

35 WHO. Primary Health Care: Report of the International Conference on Primary Health Care, Alma-Ata, USSR, 6–12 September, 1978. www.who.int/hpr/NPH/docs/declaration_almaata.pdf

36 Bender DE, Pitkin K. Bridging the gap: The village health worker as the cornerstone of the primary health care model. *Social Science and Medicine* 1987; 24:515–528.

37 Hillman D, Hillman E, Mukelebai K. *The Primary Health Care Manual for East Africa.* New York: UNICEF, 1996.

38 Hall JJ, Taylor R. Health for all beyond 2000: The demise of the Alma-Ata Declaration and primary health care in developing countries. *Medical Journal of Australia* 2003; 178:17–20.

39 Preston SA. Causes and consequences of mortality decline in less developed countries during the Twentieth Century. In RA Easterlin (ed), *Population and Economic Change in Developing Countries.* Chicago: University of Chicago Press, 1980, pp. 289–360.

40 Pritchett L, Summers LH. Wealthier is healthier. *Journal of Human Resources* 1996; 31:841–868.

41 Bloom DE, Canning D. The health and wealth of nations. *Science* 2000; 287:1207–1209.

42 www.military.com/NewsContent/0,13319,FL_cost_111804,00.html?ESRC=eb.n (last accessed: 7 May 2007).

43 Donkin A, Goldblatt P, Lynch K. Inequalities in life expectancy by social class 1972–1999. *Health Statistics Quarterly* 2002; 15:5–15.

44 Barker DJP. *Mother, Babies and Disease in Later Life,* 2nd ed. Edinburgh: Churchill Livingstone, 1998.

45 Kawachi I, Berkman L (eds). *Neighborhoods and Health.* Oxford: Oxford University Press, 2003.

46 Claussen B, Davey Smith G, Thelle D. Impact of childhood and adulthood socio-economic position on cause specific mortality: The Oslo Mortality Study. *Journal of Epidemiology and Community Health* 2003; 57:40–45.

47 Sampson RJ, Raudenbush SW, Earls F. Neighbourhoods and violent crime: A multilevel study of collective efficacy. *Science* 1997; 277:918–924.

48 Wilkinson R, Marmot M (eds). *Social Determinants of Health: The Solid Facts,* 2nd ed. Copenhagen: WHO, 2003.

49 Malthus T. *An Essay on the Principles of Population as It Affects the Future Improvement of Society.* London: Printed for J. Johnson, 1798.

50 U.N. Population Projections. Medium Projection, World. esa.un.org/unpp/ (last accessed 23 Jan. 2008).

51 The Sphere Project. www.sphereproject.org (last accessed 7 May 2007).

2 An Individual's Role

I was standing there in a mask and scrubs waiting for the surgeon to come in and start the operation. I was fresh out of medical school and doing my first international rotation in Ghana. He walked in precisely 15 minutes late. 'So have you read the operation for today?' he asked me. I nodded an affirmative yes. He said, 'Here's the scalpel. Let's get started.'

Behind the sweat and my knees knocking, I looked at the surgeon and said I was barely qualified to hold a retractor, never mind do surgery. I was a family medicine doctor, not a surgeon. To be honest, I felt like I was about to hurl. If I had to do this every day, it might be my last.

– Story told by a family medicine doctor to medical students interested in global health

A career in global health and medicine is a noble pursuit. It may begin with the best of intentions, such as wanting to help disadvantaged populations or to provide faith-based services to others. An adventurous person may also want to learn about another culture, to explore an exciting new world, to test new skills learned in medicine or epidemiology, to seek one's cultural heritage, or to learn a new language. In many cases, the motivation to pursue an international experience will be a combination of the various reasons given above. However, the reasons behind why you are choosing to have a global health experience will shape your options and future career path.

As the remainder of this guidebook will present information for more common or traditional global health experiences and careers, this chapter explores some alternative choices and unconventional pathways in global health. No matter what the career pathway may be, it is important to gain experience in developing countries or resource-poor settings, early and often. Even if you're a foreign affairs specialist writing international policy papers behind a desk, good policies must be intermixed with practical experiences 'in the field.' The stories in this chapter are about real people and real lives. They describe how several people, who do not all have a traditional background in global health, came to shape global health in unconventional but meaningful ways.

Case 1 – Do Something!

Adrian Bradbury is not your typical development specialist. He didn't go to Africa as a child. He wasn't immersed in global development issues at the University of Ottawa. As Adrian said, 'I couldn't name you one single group who was involved in global development at the University.' In school, he played varsity basketball in Ottawa and became a sports journalist.

'How did you get involved?' we asked.

Adrian blames his involvement on his 6- and 4-year-old children. 'When I had kids, I read the newspaper more and become aware of global issues. I was involved in reporting on sports, but there's only so many "give a 110%" quotes one can write about.'

So Adrian became involved in volunteering. First, he volunteered with OXFAM, by attending small events and helping with the War Child project by providing some media consulting. However, the gnawing question for him was, 'How could I do something different?'

People said he should get athletes involved.

As a sports journalist, Adrian noticed two distinct patterns by which athletes became involved. First, they did things that were very local, such as the Boys and Girls Clubs. The second way was to export sport to other countries. A third less common way was using their status as a platform to talk about real issues. For example, the two-time National Basketball Association Most Valuable Player Steve Nash has done so with his stance on peace building. Adrian realized that it was important to find key athletes, such as Steve Nash, who not only could talk about the global issues but also recruit other prominent athletes to promote dialogue about real-world issues.

With this concept in mind, Adrian started Athletes for Africa in 2003. He visited numerous non-governmental organizations (NGOs) around Toronto to learn about establishing and successfully operating his own NGO. The goal of Athletes for Africa is to raise money and awareness for the problems of Africa. It partnered with leading NGOs in Africa, including Engineers without Borders, the African Medical and Research Foundation (AMREF), and the Canadian Physicians for Aid and Relief (CPAR). By the end of 2004, while also working full-time at the University of Toronto, Adrian obtained charitable status for Athletes for Africa.

Adrian's colleagues at AMREF and CPAR told him about the plight of children in northern Uganda. Adrian searched the Internet and learned more about Uganda's problems. While he was reading *Terry: The Life of Canadian Terry Fox* by Douglas Coupland one evening, Adrian understood the importance of physically telling a story.

Adrian learned that Ugandan children walked 12.5 kilometres (8 miles) to the town of Gulu every night in order to avoid being captured by the nefarious Lord's Resistance Army (LRA), which would force them into the militia. The long walks have been common for many of the northern Ugandan children during their ongoing 20-year-old civil war. Adrian couldn't believe that over 40,000 children made the walk to town each and every day. He decided the best way to learn about their struggle was to replicate the walk that the children were doing on a daily basis.

Adrian enlisted his friend Kieran Howard and they decided if Ugandan children had to walk 8 miles every night, then they could do the same walk for just one month. In July 2005 Adrian and Kieran walked 8 miles to Toronto City Hall every night for 31 nights, starting the phenomenon now known as *GuluWalk* (www.guluwalk.com). Each night they would sleep in front of city hall to raise public and government awareness of the issue in Uganda. Then, after only 4 hours sleep, just like the children of northern Uganda, they would walk 8 miles to home. They tried to maintain their full-time jobs. In total, Adrain and Kieran walked 775 kilometres (485 miles) on mostly paved roads, and it took them 154 hours and 18 minutes over the 31 days.

Adrian and Kieran quickly realized that they couldn't live their lives like the children of northern Uganda. Adrian and Kieran made a conscious decision not to publicize their walk until 1 July, the first day of their month. Writing in a blog and diary, they received front-page attention in the *Toronto Star* by their sixth day. By their tenth day, they were receiving 150 daily e-mails. When they started, Kieran knew that the Toronto media would pick up the story. What he didn't realize was that their walk would become a national and international phenomenon. Recalling the events, Adrian said, 'The story was easy to tell and it was visual, so the media could understand. The key behind it was it was two white middle-class guys, who 80% of Toronto can relate to, sleeping in front of City Hall. You have to remember that most people have seen documentaries on Africa and aren't interested in another story on Africa. The key was how to break through the general fatigue, and the white middle-class guys doing something different was a story ... When I started, I had never touched foot in Africa, and here I was now an "expert" on Africa. It was quite strange.'

In 2006 GuluWalk enlisted Steve Nash, Lieutenant-General Romeo Dallaire (who headed the U.N. mission in Rwanda during the 1994 genocide), Sarah McLachlan (famous singer), and Chantal Kreviazuk (another famous singer) in their efforts to raise funds for the children of northern Uganda. They raised over $500,000 for the Ugandan children. The second GuluWalk occurred on 21 October 2006 in 82 cities and 15 countries. The third GuluWalk occurred on 20 October 2007 in 100 cities and 15 countries and raised another $500,000.

'The key behind GuluWalk is that each GuluWalk is a local story. It isn't about two white middle-class guys from Toronto ... but this university group from Cardiff,' explained Adrian.

Adrian believes the single most important thing for young adults getting involved in global development is to 'Do something!' It doesn't matter what that something might be, but it's more than signing online petitions or taking a passive role in trusting that problems will be solved.

Nowadays, Adrian is regularly asked to talk to groups and governments on the plight of the children in northern Uganda. He has visited the projects that GuluWalk supports. He also privately notes that he loves doing the advocacy work, though the nitty-gritty of running an organization and managing a growing operation isn't necessarily what he'd choose to do, if given the option.

But Adrain does have some sage advice for those starting in global health and development: 'Youth should be willing to challenge and advocate and "be jaded" enough to force change to occur. Think about the genocide convention and the claim by the U.S. that Darfur is genocide. If we have a convention that implies we should act and we say these events occur, why aren't we acting? Development is like a game, and the stars and athletes want to be on the playing field with the spectators cheering them on, so that they seem to be doing the right thing. However, the challenge is to bring more people from the stands down into the field.'

Adrian's final advice is 'Don't be afraid to take risks.'

Although Adrian and Kieran have never lived in the war-torn area of northern Uganda, they realized that even ordinary white middle-class men with a little bit of care (and a lot of sleepless nights) could push ideas through the right channels and make a difference in children's lives half a world away.

Case 2 – A Special Place

When Kyra Abbott was 7 year old, she witnessed the images of the Ethiopian famine on television. 'When I grow up, I want to make a difference,' she vowed. Yet, Kyra was born in Perth, a small town outside Ottawa, Canada. As she said, 'I was raised in a very small, Anglo-Saxon, homogeneous town and thus had little opportunity to pursue my interest in global health until I went away and began my university studies.'

Nursing was Kyra's opportunity to help the poor and the sick, and to go abroad, since nursing is required everywhere. The other reason that Kyra chose to enter the nursing field was that it could equip her to practise the profession with only four years of schooling 'and I was not keen to spend more years in the classroom than were absolutely necessary.'

School was where Kyra found an introduction into the field of aid, development, and global health, where she was provided with networking opportunities. Whenever possible, she was keen to learn about things 'global.'

Before entering her fourth year of university, she travelled to Zimbabwe on the International Seminar program with World University Service of Canada (WUSC) (www.wusc.ca). There, Kyra participated in several development-related workshops, conducted research on the social stigma of HIV/AIDS, and volunteered at a preschool for children of parents living with AIDS. However, Kyra's original impression was that she was very unwelcome. As she said, 'Understandably, years of oppression by white colonialists had left the nation bitter and resentful of white people in general. For me, I would not choose to work in a country where I did not feel at least accepted and hopefully welcomed by the local population.'

When Kyra graduated from nursing school, she wanted to go abroad. A summer camp colleague and friend had volunteered in Haiti with an organization that operated a large orphanage and the country's main pediatric hospital. Her friend's enthusiasm towards Haiti and its people and his positive recommendation of the organization convinced Kyra to take the plunge.

'Wow!' was the first impression Kyra had of Haiti. 'I was over-whelmed,' she said. 'Everything was so different from back home and the need was so great. The poverty was overwhelming. People were very poor and many could not afford even basic health care. Many of the children at our hospital only arrived when they were close to death.' Kyra was and continues to be very impressed by how the nurses and doctors are able to improvise and make due with the medications and materials they have available to them. '*Nothing* is wasted – a stark contrast compared to the amount of material waste in the health care system back home.' Kyra remembers thinking that she was stepping back in time – there was very limited technology in the hospitals and clinics, often without electricity and/or running water. Gravity IV infusions were something she had never experienced in Canada. Traction was applied using water jugs or rocks as weights. Kyra was also shocked at the lack of available pain medications.

When Kyra arrived at an orphanage on one of her trips to Haiti, she was horrified by what she saw. There were children without diapers peeing on plastic bed covers. Three to four children lay in each bed. Many children looked as though they hadn't been cleaned for days. But children were children and they simply wanted to play. So she played with the children and learned Creole from them, and it wasn't long until she fell in love with Haiti.

Kyra loves working with children, both abroad and at home. 'I chose to work with children because I interact with them so well,' she said. 'It is a gift I have been given, whether I am dealing with a sick child or a healthy child. Although caring for children – especially sick children – can be heartbreaking and challenging, I just love and admire their innocence and candour and joy and strength. Children are also very vulnerable and deserve special attention and care, especially in resource-poor countries where the will and good intention of their parents is often not enough to provide for their basic needs. Children are special and fragile and I want to do all I can to help them.'

Kyra felt like she needed to tell her friends and family about the conditions of these children. She wrote a series of letters and stories. Oftentimes using her own money or money donated to her by friends, family, and acquaintances back home, Kyra regularly paid for sick children to see a local doctor, to obtain hospital care, and to receive necessary operations. After 3 months of caring for the children at the Haitian orphanage, she returned home.

But Kyra yearned to go back. And when she had enough money, she did go back. Kyra has now been travelling back and forth between Canada and Haiti for 8 years, spending on average 7 months per year in Canada and 5 months in Haiti. In Canada, she worked at the Children's Hospital of Eastern Ontario and at a Community Health Centre in downtown Ottawa, which caters to a large immigrant and homeless population. Her nursing work in Canada helps pay the bills and allows her time to raise awareness of her work and the people who have touched her in Haiti, and also allows her time to generate funds to offset such costs as airfare and travel insurance. It also helps her to gain valuable clinical experience in a controlled, 'best practice' setting. And her time in Haiti brings absolute joy and meaning to her life. In Haiti, she has worked as a staff nurse, an educator, and a 'surrogate mother' at the pediatric hospital (www.nphamigos.org). Her role as 'surrogate mother' was to accompany Haitian children to the United States or the Dominican Republic for medical care that was not available in Haiti. For example, she spent 2 months in the Dominican Republic with a 3-year-old boy who had radiation treatment for retinoblastoma, a cancer of the eye. Kyra has also worked as a coordinator for a busy surgical unit at a mission hospital, as a designer and implementer of a rural kwashiorkor treatment program with a public health organization (www.haitianhealthfoundation.org), as a nurse at a small orphanage (www.haitichildren.net), and with Médecins sans Frontières (MSF) on an emergency and exploratory mission after former President Aristide fled the country (www.msf.ca).

Kyra recently began working as the Program Development and Sustainability Officer for the Healthy Mothers–Healthy Babies Foundation, a small American health-based NGO (www.hm-hb.org), which operates a rural birthing home and community health and malaria programs.

'What joys and frustrations do you have in Haiti?' Kyra was asked.

'The frustrations I have in Haiti are plenty, and the degree to which they bother me varies from day to day, week to week.' As a white person in Haiti, Kyra states that it is difficult to blend in with the masses. It is next to impossible to purchase anything in the market or off the street for the local price. She notes that to the regular Haitian, all foreigners are rich and should be 'exploited.' Although it frustrates her, she tries not to become too angry about this perception because she realizes that there is an element of truth in it. 'Although I am not rich back home and although I was not getting paid in Haiti, I still have monetary and material resources available to me.' She is one of very few foreigners who gets around via public transport and who dares to walk in the street. 'I only do so when the political situation is calm enough – but it can be hard having the other foreigners and the bourgeois [upper-class] Haitians look at you with disbelief and sometimes disdain.'

Haiti is more stable now than it has been in years, partly because of the large presence of U.N. peacekeepers. But in the past, there have certainly been periods where Kyra felt afraid to walk in the streets of Port-au-Prince because of the high incidence of kidnappings. Haiti's police force is plagued with many challenges, including corruption, lack of training, and lack of equipment. She said, 'My most frightening experience in Haiti involved a police officer. It is somewhat disconcerting and discomforting to know that if you have a problem, the police are not the people you would first turn to or could necessarily expect assistance from.'

Other frustrations Kyra has experienced include the challenges of working in an environment where resources are so limited and realizing how unfair and unjust our world is.

The biggest challenges I have faced in my international work include being unable to access the necessary medications and treatments, and coming to terms with the gross injustices that exist in health care available between the rich and poor countries. There are many barriers to accessing medication and treatments – availability, price, proper means for transportation and storage, lack of education, lack of diagnostic materials, etc. I have seen children die from asthma and pneumonia because there was no concentrated oxygen available for them. I have seen newborns die from neonatal tetanus infections because their mothers were not vaccinated. I have seen a mother bleed to death after giving birth because there was neither surgical care available nor any means of transfusing blood. I have seen people of all ages suffer with agonizing pain – from broken bones, cancer, lacerations, post-surgery – because there was only the most basic of pain medications available. I have seen many children and adults die because they could not access the tuberculosis or antiretroviral medications they so desperately needed.

Kyra also explained that it is challenging for her to return to Canada and to reintegrate into the health care field there, 'where technology and treatments are so advanced, where there are many wasted resources, and many dissatisfied health care recipients. Although I realize this subject is very sensitive and controversial, I often feel that at home we invest exorbitant and unnecessary amounts of financial and human resources to keep people alive because we refuse to let go, we are afraid of death. Too often the gift to die peacefully and naturally with dignity should be chosen but is not. Whereas in Haiti (and other poor countries), people die needlessly and en masse from preventable and treatable illnesses, because the basic necessary resources are just not available.'

As Kyra pointed out, the joys of working in Haiti are plentiful or she would not have returned. She asserts that it is the relationships and human interactions that she most enjoys:

With my patients and their families, with my co-workers, and with regular people on the street, like the lady who sells me my daily banana. Respecting others and having that respect reciprocated. And there is a raw beauty in sharing in another's suffering and hardship – suffering with them, just being there and providing support. There is satisfaction at a very basic level of simply being present and doing what you can. No matter whether the outcome is positive or negative, people appreciate that you have come from far away and that you have tried to do something – that you have not forgotten them. It is these basic interactions that are so real and so human that inspire me to keep doing this type of work. Of course it is also wonderful to see children recover from illnesses after assuming they would most certainly die because they were so sick and the resources available to care for them so basic. To have children run after you and smile and smother you with hugs and shout with glee is wonderful too!

Kyra's advice is:

Go for it! There are a million opportunities out there – paid and unpaid, short term and long term, far away and close to home. My first experience in a resource-poor country [Zimbabwe] was nothing like what I had expected – I was disappointed, disheartened, and discouraged. But then I travelled to another country and fell in love with its people and culture. The world is big and the needs are great – I wish everyone would spend part of their career helping those who are less fortunate, wherever they may be. I would remind people of the importance of observation and understanding. No one likes or respects the newcomer who arrives and immediately criticizes the current situation and practices. Change takes time. There may be a good reason they are doing things the way they are. Remember that you are simply passing through. Often you will learn more and get more from your experience than you can possibly give.

What does the future hold for Kyra?

Shortly after graduation, Kyra enrolled in several courses in Seneca College's International Health program and has now almost completed a post-graduate Certificate in International Development from the University of British Columbia via distance education. She will soon begin a post-graduate Certificate in International Development Management from Humber College.

When asked where she might like to end up, Kyra replied, 'I'd like to continue working in the global health field. I feel that my background in nursing and now my studies in international development and international development management should enable me to be a competent and capable project coordinator. I would like to continue working in the non-profit industry, sometimes based in Canada and often based "in the field."'

Case 3 – Telling a Story

Linda Harrar is an award-winning independent producer who specializes in documentaries with a human perspective on science and technology, nature, and society. She was a staff producer on the NOVA series for 12 years, and was the first producer to document the hole in the Antarctic ozone layer.

For a long time, Linda was interested in global health, after doing a documentary on children's survival in the 1980s. Furthermore, her interests and documentaries were clearly focused on the environment and health.

In the fall of 2001, Linda approached Paula Apsell, senior editor for NOVA at the Public Broadcasting Service (PBS), and Richard Hutton, the vice-president of Vulcan Productions, to create a documentary called *Rx for Survival*, which was being funded by the Bill and Melinda Gates Foundation. The Bill and Melinda Gates Foundation wanted an additional component, which was an impact campaign. After approval, the Merck Foundation also joined on-board to help fund the project.

Linda reflected on why she accepted the production of *Rx for Survival*, saying: 'One of the things that was exciting in doing *Rx for Survival* was that it provided an opportunity to tell a story about the stories of individuals in circumstances of struggle. We could place historical [global health] events over time, and show changes. The key is we had the opportunity to tell powerful stories and engage people that wouldn't be reached otherwise.'

Over the next 2 years Linda and her team led by Larry Klein, who was the executive producer, met with the leaders of the global health movement. They looked for broad global health themes, from malaria to vaccinations, such as smallpox and polio. They looked at historical, events and breakthroughs in health that led to significant global health changes from the discovery of vaccination to germ theory, to John Snow's discovery of cholera.

They decided to film six different episodes, each with an individual producer, cameraman, and assistant around the world. Starting in February 2003, until its production in the fall of 2005, they travelled to different countries to document the plight of the world's poorest and most unfortunate people. Linda said, 'The key is how do you tell powerful stories. As someone once said, a single death is a tragedy. A million deaths is a statistic. The key in great filmmaking is to move the audience and to engage them powerfully in the stories themselves.'

Linda highlights an important fact in telling a story – the need to recognize the audience. In fact, the best stories are ones in which individuals are finding large obstacles, and how individuals find their way around these big problems. One of the great barriers, especially with people dying, is that they need to trust you to let you into their lives, in a precious moment.

There are barriers to filmmaking, like there are to doing global development. One of the crews wanted to film the last person with smallpox in Somalia, but the in-country people known as 'fixers' weren't sure about security. In the end, they decided not to film in Somalia for that simple reason.

One of the exciting parts of the project was the impact campaign that worked with partners, Save the Children and CARE, to help people learn about global health. Its aim was not to be a lobbying group for global health, but to open channels of communication with ordinary citizens on global health. The focus was on highlighting a package of essential child health interventions and to help fundraise, from which most of the proceeds went to UNICEF.

If there is one regret, Linda wished it could have been a larger series and for *Rx for Survival* to have been tied more closely with the impact campaign. However, Linda believes there is an important role for good journalism and reporting related to global health issues. She wants to report not only the 'bad ill effects of health,' but also some of the creative solutions that have been implemented to address some of the global health problems.

Linda said: 'We need to engage the public and the audience about the issues. If there is one thing I can be satisfied with, it's that *Rx for Survival* has led to many e-mails and phone calls about people changing professions, and changing directions into global health. Everything from funding malaria bed nets to volunteering abroad. We need to encourage more Americans to get involved in things outside our own borders.'

Case 4 – Hearing the Voices of Children

In 1985, 27-year-old soon-to-be lawyer Peter Dalglish, while articling in Halifax, Canada, was watching a television program showing starving children in Ethiopia and Somalia. He had an epiphany; he wanted to do something to help those destitute children. Peter bought a one-way ticket to Khartoum. After he arrived, Peter just couldn't believe the scope of the starvation and poverty he was seeing in Africa. Peter wanted to help. He then obtained a position as the coordinator of the emergency unit with the World Food Program (WFP) in Darfur, Western Sudan, along the desert border between Chad and Sudan. It was a massive responsibility trying to find food for 50,000 displaced children.

Peter quickly learned from colleagues at the Red Cross and Médecins sans Frontières (Doctors without Borders) about the methods behind transporting supplies to the front lines. The conversations and the stories with these front-line workers changed his attitudes towards humanitarian workers. He also learned quickly about the need to 'find a mentor.' These included colleagues who were similar to him in age, such as Alex de Waal, then of Save the Children, who had had significant on-the-ground experience. Other more-seasoned mentors included Cole Dodge, who worked in East Africa in northern Uganda, and Richard Jolly, the architect of UNICEF's work on 'Adjustment with a Human Face' and his ground-breaking work on founding the Human Development Report. One of Peter's favourite mentors was Alec Dickson, a founder of Volunteer Services Overseas (VSO), whose words of encouragement to young mentors were simply, 'You are needed.'

The first 3 months were spent looking for local *souks* (markets) and seeking camels to transport supplies to the refugee camps along the Chad–Sudan border. He remembers seeing young girls and boys selling empty food grain bags with the words 'A Gift from the People of the United States of America.'

In Khartoum, one evening in May 1985, Peter returned to his Toyota

Land Cruiser and saw a 10-year-old Sudanese boy trying to break into it using a bent nail. Peter grabbed the boy. The boy stood terrified.

'No, I'm not here to hurt you,' Peter said.

Instead, he gave the boy some food. The boy ate the food hungrily, and then asked for more. Peter realized the enormous talent of the young child. Peter went to the streets to learn more about these children. He discovered that they had little to do other than steal in order to get food. He knew that without opportunities and hope these children would continue stealing and in the end be left with nothing.

Peter decided, with some help from rocker Bob Geldof (of Live Aid fame), to start the first technical training school for street children. He helped turn the street kids into mechanics, welders, and electricians. His students were soon hired by local businesses. Peter then started a same-day courier service for businesses that was run by the street kids, and it also flourished.

Fresh from these successes in Africa, Peter returned to Canada in 1987 and founded Street Kids International (SKI) with nothing more than a desk, a telephone, and the hope of bringing similar projects to street children in countries around the world. His organization went to the National Film Board and fundraised 2 million dollars (Can). Then, they helped develop innovative programs, including an animated film to educate street kids about AIDS and street drugs, which has won awards and gained worldwide attention including the Peter Drucker Award for Innovation.

'It was a small organization with brilliant ideas and it worked, because it didn't require 50 people,' Peter said.

One of the most important aspects was that SKI wasn't afraid to test the boundaries, including teaming up with the private sector. This approach allowed for more innovation. However, at the same time, Peter was acutely aware of 'founder's syndrome' – the need for founders to remain in control of their organization and their ideas. He was also acutely aware of a founder's visionary nature, but also of being difficult when it came to changing with ideas and being perhaps a poor manager as a whole. So to allow SKI to grow, Peter felt that he had to leave the organization so that it could foster and explore new avenues.

Peter became executive secretary of Youth Services Jeunesse, which works with out-of-school and out-of-work Canadian youth, and allows them to take charge of their direction and map their own initiatives. While there, he viewed the importance of services by youth, such as advocated by John McKnight at Northwestern University in Chicago, which promoted asset-based community development.

Over the past 5 years, Peter has worked as the chief technical adviser on child labour to the International Labour Organization in Nepal. One of his challenges has been to change an institutional approach to caring for children, which emphasized orphanages over family care. Working with the Red Cross and Save the Children, Peter spearheaded this initiative to bring children back to the family. A second initiative was to treat children affected by HIV/AIDS. A third was to allow more apprenticeship training for young children.

Finally, Peter has worked a lot on anti-trafficking of children from Nepal to India. 'Often, children who work in drug trafficking are picked up by police and placed into detention,' he said. 'Do you know what they do when they get out? They go into prostitution ... Very rarely do they return home.' As Peter went on to say, there are three challenging questions that NGOs working in this arena need to ask: 'First, do they want to be rescued? Second, do they want to be rescued by you? Finally, where are they now?'

There are often significant challenges with working in developing countries. Sometimes, it's important to navigate politics, but at the heart of getting things done is the need to establish strong relationships with credible individuals. It's also important to protect people who are key in getting things done.

Peter also founded Schools without Borders, an organization whose goal is to facilitate opportunities for privileged youth in Canada to work with disadvantaged populations overseas. It aims to provide life experiences, from ships off Holland and learning with leading social entrepreneurs and environmental workers. One of the fun initiatives that Schools without Borders has participated in is working with the NGO, Viva Rio, which brings workers from the flavellas in Rio to teach students about social justice and developing a moral conscience. Peter told us:

> At the end of the day, I look at the statistics from my graduating class at Stanford [1979]. Do you know that the average person in my graduating class makes U.S. $210,000, and has probably less than three weeks of vacation a year. When I ask them what they do to make the world a better place, they talk about donating money to a charity, or working with their church, mosque or synagogue ... However, what I do is immensely rewarding and it's a privilege to be let into the lives of street children.

If there's one word of advice: 'Start young.' When I look into the eyes of a student who comes to me and tells me that [he or she] wants to make some money and then come back to help, I know they won't be back. Their lives and their comforts take over.

It's this passion for helping the child without a voice that makes Peter unique. His moral compass shows us the direction we can take to make a difference. More than anything, Peter displays a moral conscience. With a little ingenuity, no matter what background or academic degree a person may have, anyone can make a difference.

Case 5 – A Life of Joy

In 1969, Drs Elizabeth 'Liz' and Donald 'Don' Hillman, both practising pediatricians, were asked to join a Canadian International Development Agency (CIDA) academic program at McGill University. Their role was to support a new medical school at the University of Nairobi in Kenya, as Kenyan students previously had to go to Makerere University in Uganda to study medicine. Their mentor, Dr Alan Ross, asked them to help establish the McGill–Kenya CIDA program.

Liz and Don didn't hesitate. They packed up their five children, whose ages ranged from 3 to 12, and travelled to East Africa. There was no hesitation in bringing the children. Liz said, 'We enjoy our children and learn from them. Children make you instantly a part of the African community.' There aren't any problems with children as long as you do the sensible things, like wash your hands, eat sensibly, and be careful. But the opportunities exist to work with your children as a team to learn all about healthy behaviours, cultural events, and wonderful opportunities.

'None of our five children had serious illness except one who was written up as the first *mzungu* (white person) who contracted dengue on the coast of Kenya!'

When they arrived in Kenya, there was no pediatrics department. They asked if they could have some clinical space to see children. In a small little abandoned building, along with Dr Ross, Liz and Don put together beds and built a space where they could provide medical care to sick children. They established a clinical service of pediatrics and helped shape the teaching hospital by placing pediatrics as an important core component of the medical curriculum.

Liz and Don soon realized that many of the children were being brought in by sick mothers, who themselves were not receiving adequate medical care. They knew the children wouldn't get better without also taking care of their mothers. From their observations, they decided their focus should not be solely on the children, but had to also include the mothers. Liz and Don became the early proponents of the maternal–child health dyad, a tenet of modern global health that considers the health of a child to be related to the health of his or her mother. Liz and Don took medical residents from McGill University to Nairobi and its surrounding communities in order to show them the challenges that Kenyans faced on a daily basis. Liz and Don taught the students and medical community that delivery of health care isn't just about medicine; it's also about the social, political, and economic determinants that affect an individual's health. However, the residents benefited as well, because as Liz said, 'Residents are the best teachers and did a marvellous job over the 10 years the McGill project lasted.'

Liz and Don had two separate stints in Kenya. Their first stint was from 1969 to 1971, and their second stint was also spent at the University of Nairobi, as field directors of the McGill–CIDA program from 1974 to 1976.

After several years in Kenya, Liz and Don returned to Canada, to Memorial University in St John's, Newfoundland, where Liz became the Head of Ambulatory Medicine and Don became the chair of the Department of Pediatrics. During this time, they were asked to help rebuild the Pediatrics Department at Makerere University in Uganda. After they accepted the challenge, Don was named physician-in-chief of Makerere University.

As they recalled, shaping Makerere University was an extremely difficult challenge, in part because there was a severe shortage of physicians to teach at the medical school. The country had been recently ruled by Idi Amin, so there were also political and military challenges. 'We came to a school that had holes, bullets, and constant gunfire,' Don said.

Don and Liz submitted a report that led to the creation of the Child Health and Medical Education Program (CHAMP), which helped the development, assessment, and expansion of primary health care in Kenya, Uganda, Zambia, and Tanzania. The program was well received in Uganda, and it helped rebuild links to other parts of the country, and eventually culminated in the development of the Makerere Child Health and Development Center. The Center brought together community, government, and university interests.

As part of these initiatives, Liz and Don continued to link universities throughout East Africa. Since colleagues in neighbouring countries were facing similar child health problems, it made sense to collaborate with similar universities in Nairobi, Kenya, Dar es Salaam, Tanzania, and Lusaka, Zambia. Together, they worked on joint initiatives to promote teaching, service, and research of primary health care, and to bring the brightest, young leaders interested in global child health. Building these East African–led initiatives through the universities was extremely important to Liz and Don, because they could share research and learning plans, how to measure progress, and best methods. The collaboration grew from four to eight and then 12 universities through East Africa. At the same time, partnerships and colleagues from 12 of 16 Canadian universities went to work with CHAMP partners in Africa to help in teaching and measuring progress.

Universities are a special place for Liz and Don, as universities have great student leaders who have the best ideas and the time to carry them out. 'Students have always been the most important part of our lives.'

To Liz and Don, primary health care has a very basic social definition. When Liz first went into the community with her students to ask about their health priorities, the community pointed to a big pile of trash. So, that's what her medical students did; they picked up the trash. When the communities saw what a marvellous job the medical students did cleaning the garbage, they were more willing to talk about the traditional definitions of health.

At the end of their time in Uganda, Liz and Don returned to Canada to help create the Centre for International Health at McMaster University and the Centre for International Health and Development at the University of Ottawa. During their 'retirement,' Liz and Don continue to work on over 20 different global health projects while still finding time to inspire numerous medical students, residents, and faculty members to get involved in global health and medicine.

Liz highlighted three lessons to take from global health and medicine:

1 Look at your personal reason for working internationally. Be honest.
2 Listen and learn from your colleagues who have been successful in their involvement globally. Why did it work for them?
3 Know the place you are going to. Read, listen, learn, and be ready to share *your* strength in the partnership you develop. Keep in contact with your international partners. Use what you learn from them in your own practice, which becomes more international every year.

The following three things stand out about Liz and Don's story: the absolute joy they bring in all things they do, the importance they place on family and friends as a priority above their global health work, and their incredible bond as a couple in everything they do together. They prove that global health isn't something that one has to do alone or while excluding a family. In fact, they proved quite the opposite to be true. Experiencing another culture and living abroad with someone you love or with a family can be very compatible with working in global health and medicine.

Since the original interview was conducted, Donald Hillman unfortunately succumbed to pneumonia. His presence in global health will sorely be missed.

Case 6 – Believing in Water

Ryan Hreljac was 6 years old and a first-grader when he heard that children in Africa were dying because they had no access to clean water. 'How could that be?' he thought. There was clean water from every tap in his house. He was bothered by the simple fact that the African children could die from drinking their unclean water. He did some research and discovered that constructing a new water well would cost $70.

At first, he begged his parents for $70. They said, 'We'll think about it,' hoping that Ryan would forget about the matter. Ryan didn't forget, and he kept asking day after day. His parents had him do chores to earn the $70. After 4 months, Ryan had $70, enough money to build one new water well for some children in Africa. Ryan proudly went to an organization that builds water wells in Africa, and he gave them his jar of money containing $70.

Unfortunately, the organization told him the cost of a new water well was not $70, but $2,000. Instead of being crestfallen, Ryan decided that he would do more chores. Then, a local reporter heard about Ryan and his goal, and printed his story in a local newspaper. People started sending Ryan cheques for various amounts: $25 here, $20 there.

Soon, a newspaper from the nearby city heard about Ryan, and they printed his story in their newspaper. Ryan quickly had the $2,000 he needed to pay for building a new water well in Africa. Then, Ryan heard that for $25,000 he could buy a drill that could build many water wells. A local water well builder read the story and donated $2,000 to Ryan. Soon, Ryan had raised $25,000.

WaterCan, the organization that accepted Ryan's donation, decided it was time to build Ryan's new water well in Uganda. Ryan asked that his water well be built near a school, so the children would have access to clean water. Just before construction started on the water well, Ryan started receiving letters from a pen pal in Uganda named Jimmy Akana.

By this time, *Reader's Digest* decided to publish a story on Ryan and his quest to build water wells in Uganda. A film crew from a Canadian television station accompanied Ryan on his trip to Uganda. The cover story in the *Reader's Digest* and the subsequent documentary of Ryan's trip made him a national celebrity.

But for Ryan, the opportunity to meet his new friend, Jimmy Akana, in Uganda was a highlight. Oprah Winfrey saw the cover of *Reader's Digest* and invited the boy to her show. Overnight, thousands of dollars came in to support Ryan's quest to build clean water systems in Africa.

Over the past 7 years, Ryan has raised millions of dollars and helped fund the construction of over 150 water wells in Africa. He has won numerous international awards including the Child of the World prize. Incidentally, when he learned that the other finalist for the Child of the World prize, a boy from Brazil, wasn't receiving the $15,000 cash prize, Ryan offered to share it with him. Upon hearing of Ryan's offer, the founder of the award decided to give both boys the $15,000 prize.

The story doesn't end here. In 2003 Ryan and his family heard that the Lord's Resistance Army in northern Uganda had captured Jimmy Akana. However, Jimmy had escaped and was staying with a friend of his family. Ryan and his family, with some help from friends, eventually flew Jimmy to Canada, where he was granted asylum and eventually refugee status. Jimmy Akana was adopted by Ryan's family, and he now lives with them in Canada.

Ryan's story is special. It shows that no matter how young, how small, and how unfathomable the challenge of global health may be, we can all raise awareness of important global health issues and make a difference.

3 Understanding the Landscape and Identifying Your Goals

Many people say something along the lines of 'I would like to do something in global health, but I don't know how to get started.' Maybe you are saying something similar. Becoming involved in global health is not difficult once you understand the global health landscape and identify your goals. There are many different areas of global health and medicine, and thus many different ways to become engaged. While opportunities within nearly all of these areas have been expanding in recent years, some areas of global health have had more rapid growth than others. This has been in large part due to trends in funding from governmental and non-governmental organizations (NGOs). The landscape of global health should constantly evolve in order to keep up with the changes in knowledge and experience, as well as the needs and demands of people in developing countries.

People often want to move quickly in contacting several organizations in hopes of finding their ideal position in some faraway country. However, trying to find a global health experience in a haphazard manner without first understanding the basic landscape often leaves people frustrated and with the disillusion that global health is a closed society. In fact, there are many opportunities available to people with various backgrounds, education levels, and degrees of international experience. To obtain a global health experience that is most tailored to your background and interests, you should first take some time to understand the types of opportunities available. This will not only help you determine the most suitable way to become engaged, but will also help you obtain your experience more efficiently.

This chapter presents the landscape of global health from a perspective of potential opportunities and experiences. The six major areas of

Table 3.1
Six Major Areas of Global Health Opportunities

1 Research
2 Clinical Work
3 Short-Term Work
  • 'Work vacations'
  • Consulting assignments
4 Long-Term Work
5 Education
  • Language immersion course
  • Global health conference
  • Short course in tropical medicine or public health
  • Graduate training in global health-related program
6 Developing a New Project

global health opportunities are research, clinical work, short-term work, long-term work, education, and developing a new project (see Table 3.1). While global health opportunities could be categorized differently, nearly all of the global health experiences you are likely to seek or encounter can be described within these six major areas. After describing the landscape, we provide a section to help you identify your goals in global health. We provide some questions and special considerations to help you determine which type of global health experience is best suited to your interests, limitations, and motivations.

The remainder of this guidebook will be structured to help you navigate the vast array of global health opportunities according to the type of experience you are seeking. Therefore, understanding the landscape and identifying your goals will not only better prepare you to communicate your interests and ideas when approaching individuals, organizations, and programs, but will also enable you to efficiently use this guidebook.

Before describing the global health landscape, there are several issues worth addressing. First and foremost, a key element to most successful international projects and experiences has been building effective partnerships with people and institutions in developing countries. This is true for all types of international experiences, including volunteering, consulting, or learning. Establishing continuity with people or organizations will help foster a more cohesive exchange of information and resources. Therefore, as a general rule, all international work should be done in conjunction with, and not in place of, partners from the host country. Furthermore, the goal of most global health projects, if not all, is to achieve sustainable improvements in health. Sustainable changes almost always involve teaching and training local people.

Another important consideration with global health work is the impact of your presence and work. Sometimes your presence in certain situations will generate more problems than solutions. Remembering that you are a guest and knowing if and when you might need to disengage from a project or location is an important skill. In addition, not all global health work is beneficial. All projects and programs should be regularly evaluated for their impact and effects. Program evaluations could either be formal or informal, and those projects with less than favourable evaluations should either be redirected or stopped. Finally, the results of any project, favourable or not, should be shared with others. Even projects that 'fail' to achieve their goals have important lessons that are worth sharing.

Research

Research is vitally important to understanding and advancing global health issues. Much of the health-related research being conducted in developing countries relates to tropical diseases and diseases more common among the poor, including HIV/AIDS, malaria, tuberculosis, and malnutrition. Recently, increased attention to the importance of health care delivery and public health systems has invigorated research efforts on allocation and utilization of health care resources and personnel. While most health-related research being conducted in developing countries is in the realm of public health or clinical medicine, many international research opportunities exist in other health-related fields, including anthropology, geography, laboratory sciences, economics, human rights, psychology, civil engineering, sociology, and political science.

Academic institutions and pharmaceutical companies have historically conducted most of the global health research, while governmental and non-governmental organizations have focused more on program implementation. Currently, the funding agencies for global health, including government organizations and foundations, are becoming more involved in research activities. About 30 universities and their affiliated institutions, most of which are in the United States, are conducting most of the studies in developing countries, and thus are responsible for a significant portion of global health research. Much funding for international research comes from government institutions, such as the U.S. National Institutes of Health Fogarty International Center, and wealthy foundations, such as the Bill and Melinda Gates Foundation, the Wellcome Trust, the Rockefeller Foundation, and the Ford Foundation.

There are various opportunities and types of positions available in global health research. Obtaining an appropriate research position will depend on your level of training and amount of prior research experience. These positions might be located in either developed or developing countries. If you do not hold a graduate degree and have only minimal research experience, then you might seek a position working on a project of a larger study. If you hold a master's level graduate degree or have several years of research experience, then you could manage part or all of a research study and assist in publishing articles. If you hold a doctorate or have many years of experience, then you are better qualified to design research projects, apply for grant funding, supervise studies, and teach graduate-level courses.

Existing global health–related research rotations are listed in Chapter 4. Research-oriented fellowships, which are an excellent opportunity for students and those with minimal prior research experience, and funding assistance for research proposals are described in Chapter 7. Directly contacting universities and institutions to inquire about researchers can also be lucrative, and global health–oriented schools and programs are listed in Chapter 6. Finally, individuals wanting to develop an international research project, which has significant ethical considerations, are encouraged to work with the support of an academic institution or research-experienced organization.

Clinical Work

Conducting clinical work in a developing country can be a very enriching and rewarding experience. It can enhance clinical skills and knowledge of tropical diseases. Most clinical opportunities are available to those who have or are in the process of obtaining a medical or nursing degree. However, there are some opportunities available to physician assistants, allied health professionals, such as physical therapists, occupational therapists, and pharmacists, and those with technical skills, such as surgical assistants and phlebotomists. The main avenues for possible clinical opportunities include observing or participating in medical care at an established local clinic or hospital, providing health care with a non-governmental health care delivery organization, teaching about health care delivery, and establishing health care services within a developing country. While these options vary in scope and intensity, clinicians should be careful not to practise medical care outside their abilities and without appropriate local approval or licensure, which can usually be arranged through the local organization. Chapter 8 provides details on the necessity of obtaining a medical licence for clinical work in a developing country.

Many programs have been created in recent years to afford clinicians or student clinicians an opportunity to observe or participate in medical care at an established health care facility within a resource-poor setting. Many programs, but not all, are specifically tailored to fourth-year medical students or medical residents. Since medical schools and residency programs are encouraging more people to do a clinical rotation abroad and are creating more opportunities, they can often be a valuable resource for arranging international clinical work. However, opportunities can also be arranged by directly contacting a hospital or clinic in a developing country. We would recommend having the clinical rotation arranged well in advance, if possible. Since many hospitals and clinics are typically agreeable to hosting a visiting clinician, resident, or student, clinical work can often be arranged after arriving in a host country. However, you should be prepared to show some documentation of your prior or current clinical training. Furthermore, it is important that your clinical assistance doesn't further burden your hosts. While many clinical opportunities are not formally described, a number of established international medical electives can be found in Chapter 4.

Several NGOs provide health care services in developing countries. While these can be both short-term and long-term opportunities, most programs are less amenable to accept clinicians and health care workers who are still completing their training. These organizations are typically designed as mobile medical teams that can provide specialized medical services to a region or country, and the scope of work can range from performing a specific surgery to delivering primary care services in a refugee camp. For example, Operation Smile is an organization with oral surgeons who perform cleft palate repairs. By contrast, Médecins sans Frontières (Doctors without Borders) is a Nobel Peace Prize–winning organization that delivers medical services to displaced persons in refugee camps and war-torn areas around the world. However, these programs are not exclusively for physicians. They also hire logisticians, engineers, physician assistants, nurses, medical technicians, language translators, and others. These positions are often highly sought after and must be arranged before arriving at the local site. A listing of organizations that offer either short- or long-term clinical opportunities is offered in Chapter 5.

Finally, another avenue to pursue clinical work is to establish some health care services in a developing country. While more permanent services offer a more sustainable method for delivering health care, both creating and maintaining these programs entail making a long-term commitment to a particular area. Partners in Health, founded by Paul Farmer, Jim Kim, and Ophelia Dahl, is one such organization that established a health care clinic and has been providing medical services in rural Haiti. The process of establishing health care services is beyond the scope of this book. If you are interested in establishing health care services in a developing country, read the section on 'Developing a New Project' in this chapter, speak with people who have established similar services, and consult additional resources and references about health care delivery in a developing country.

Short-Term Work

After research and clinical work, working opportunities are the other major common pathway to get involved in global health. Since the types of opportunities greatly differ according to the amount of time you are able or willing to commit, short-term and long-term opportunities are described separately. Short-term experiences are opportunities that are less than 6 months, with most experiences lasting less than 2 months. The limited number of short-term work opportunities available in global health is mostly in the form of 'work vacations' and project-specific short-term assignments.

Several NGOs arrange work vacations, which are usually specific projects that can be completed by a group of five to twenty people within 2 to 3 weeks. The principal benefit of these projects is that the organization arranges all of the logistical details, including the project approval, accommodations, and transportation. These projects are often designed as annual trips to the same location. As the name implies, these projects are best suited for people who want to take vacation time to complete a global health project. In addition to volunteering time to a project, programs require participants to pay for their administrative efforts, and often the cost is not insignificant. However, if time is limited and money is less of a problem, then these experiences can be personally rewarding and highly valuable for the local communities. Habitat for Humanity is one example of an organization that has established construction-related work vacations in many resource-poor settings around the world. Non-governmental organizations that offer short-term work vacations are listed in Chapter 5.

Another option for short-term work is obtaining a position with a governmental or non-governmental organization that seeks assistance for an established project. Since organizations are generally less willing to invest much time and effort into hiring and preparing someone for a short-term assignment, these positions are usually very limited and difficult to obtain. If you have minimal training and experience, you may consider volunteering for a short-term assignment. These opportunities may be more easily arranged within a developing country, and can often lead to a paid position or a long-term assignment. If you have advanced training or significant working experience in global health, then you may be able to obtain a paid, short-term consulting position. Many of the consulting positions are obtained through professional contacts, but some may be found through direct contact with an organization. Non-governmental and governmental organizations that may accept or hire volunteers or consultants for short-term work assignments are listed in Chapter 5.

Finally, a brief word of caution and some advice on short-term work assignments, since these projects often face some criticism from the global health community. These programs are generally criticized for being too short for the participant to understand the needs of the local community or to provide adequate follow-up to ensure sustainability of the project after the participants leave. Experienced health workers often see well-intentioned development projects that have fallen into disuse because the constructors either did not use locally available materials or didn't understand the local needs of the community. Often short-term opportunities are of greatest value when the work augments the efforts of a long-term project that oversees the continuation of the program. However, not everyone has the ability to commit longer periods of time to global health work, and there are some good short-term programs and projects that can be beneficial to local communities. One of the more accepted short-term opportunities are specialized surgical teams that can improve a patient's quality of life with minimal need for further care. Before accepting one of these assignments, spending some time to assess the legitimacy of the program and its sustainable impact on the community is highly valuable.

Long-Term Work

Significantly more work opportunities exist for people who are able to devote more than 6 months to a particular project or organization. Long-term projects afford an individual time to learn the local language and customs, identify the lifestyles and culture of the people, and develop a greater appreciation for the daily life of people in a developing country. In addition, long-term projects tend to be more appropriate and sustainable for a local community. In general, not only do participants find long-term global health work to be more rewarding and enriching than short-term assignments, but they also tend to be of greater benefit to a local community.

Long-term global health work varies tremendously with the type of work, level of position, and field of global health. There are thousands of governmental and non-governmental organizations conducting a wide range of global health work, including public health program implementation and advocacy, supporting economic development, and global health advocacy. Certainly, people holding a graduate-level degree or having several years of work experience in a developing country would be better qualified to obtain a well-paying, long-term position. However, a graduate degree and relevant work experience are not necessary to obtaining a long-term position. Entry-level positions can be obtained with both governmental and non-governmental organizations. An excellent opportunity for an American to gain an introductory 2-year experience in global health is serving as a volunteer with the U.S. Peace Corps. Entry-level global health positions can also be arranged with NGOs within either a developed or developing country, but obtaining one of these positions may take some effort. Many people working in global health have a graduate degree in a global health–related field, and these people have an easier time finding employment than those without a graduate degree. However, even recent master's-level graduates may not have an easy time finding an overseas assignment. Fellowship programs, such as the Population Leadership Program, can serve as an entrance for recent graduates and may lead to a paid position within an organization. Supervisory and management positions are reserved for those with a graduate degree and significant working experience. Governmental and non-governmental organizations that offer long-term global health work are listed in Chapter 5, and long-term fellowships in global health–related fields are listed in Chapter 7.

Since many people often have difficulty obtaining their first long-term global health position, here are some suggestions. First, keep in mind that not all positions are located in developing countries. Obtaining a position in the United States or another developed country could provide a good entrance to a global health organization and may later lead to an overseas assignment. Many of the non-governmental organizations are located in Washington, DC, New York City, Seattle, Ottawa (Canada), and Geneva (Switzerland), near the headquarters of the World Health Organization. Second, one of the best ways to find a position is by networking with global health experts and organizations. Since many positions are often obtained through personal contacts, be willing to ask people if they know someone working in global health. Additional networking opportunities are available at the many global health conferences, where organizations set up informational booths, recruit for open positions, and may conduct interviews. Third, the global health field remains tight on funding, and you may be more likely to obtain a long-term position if you are first willing to volunteer your time. Finally, making yourself more marketable by obtaining further training or additional skills can often serve as a vehicle to obtain global health work. A recent college graduate will have limited, but available, opportunities, while a recent graduate with a global health–oriented master's degree in public health will be very marketable for long-term work opportunities in global health.

Another career pathway, which is extremely valuable and often overlooked, is public health and global health advocacy. Opportunities can exist with organizations focused on advocacy work, such as DATA (Debt relief, AIDS, Trade, and Africa), or a more general organization, such as Amnesty International or a local global health advocacy group. Finally, these positions are not necessarily located in developing countries, and are often good for people with more marketable skills. In finding a job or opportunity with these groups, find a passion that suits you, and then look for a suitable organization. Sometimes all you need to do is ask around in your local community.

Education

In addition to research, clinical work, and short-term and long-term work, many educational opportunities are available in global health. Obtaining additional global health knowledge can serve as an excellent way to become involved in global health while also strengthening your knowledge and bolstering your future prospects. Attending short educational courses or obtaining a graduate degree is beneficial for anyone with minimal training in global health. Educational opportunities in global health include intensive language immersion courses, global health conferences, short courses in public health or tropical medicine, and graduate training in global health–related programs.

Intensive language immersion courses have become popular in recent years as a way to learn a foreign language while being exposed to a different culture. Language courses typically last 2 to 6 weeks and are available in almost any developing country. Many programs can arrange a homestay with a local family. Some are tailored specifically to teach medical terms. Instruction may be via a group setting or one on one. In particular, Spanish language immersion courses located in Latin America have become very abundant, and they are listed in Chapter 4.

Global health conferences have become more numerous in recent years, and they offer participants an opportunity to learn more about global health topics and a chance to meet some experts and representatives of organizations. Some conferences allow organizations to have booths to highlight their projects and discuss their employment or volunteer opportunities. The largest conference devoted to global health in the United States is the annual Global Health Council conference held in Washington, DC, at the end of May or the beginning of June. Descriptions of global health conferences can be found in Chapter 4.

People wanting to learn more about global health within a limited time can take a short course on tropical medicine or global public health. These courses are a good option for someone with an advanced degree to become more familiar about a specific global health area. Many of these courses, but not all, are conducted in a developing country. The Gorgas Tropical Medicine course in Peru is one example of a well-established course for physicians to learn about tropical medicine over a 2- to 3-week period. Tulane University and the University of West Virginia also have summer courses that grant certificates in tropical medicine. Descriptions of short courses in public health and tropical medicine are listed in Chapter 4.

Finally, people with more of a commitment to global health may want to consider obtaining a graduate degree in a global health–related field. Many schools of public health offer a concentration in global health, and a few offer a doctorate-level degree in global health. Schools of medicine and nursing are continuing to offer more international opportunities. A number of residency programs offer international tracks, where residents have allocated time and funding for international clinical rotations. The University of Cincinnati Family Practice Residency Program and the St Joseph's Family Practice Residency in South Bend, Indiana, are two excellent examples. Finally, as we have previously mentioned, global health education can be obtained through a variety of departments and degree-granting programs, some of which include anthropology, geography, laboratory sciences, economics, civil engineering, sociology, and political science. A detailed listing of schools of public health, medicine, and nursing, medical residency programs, and other educational programs that have an emphasis on global health is provided in Chapter 6.

Developing a New Project

Without a doubt, it is much easier to find a position with an organization or project that is already established in a developing country than it is to create or develop a new project. However, developing a new project can be highly rewarding and beneficial, while providing a greater degree of ownership and autonomy. In some remote areas, developing a new project may be the only option. As a word of caution, creating a new project can also bring a lot of frustration, particularly in securing support from the local community and government, and it usually takes much longer to reach maturity than working through an established organization or project. As a guide, a minimal commitment for a new project is 5 years. The process of developing and establishing a new health project in a developing country is arduous and complicated, and detailing this process is beyond the scope of this guidebook. Therefore, in addition to providing a word of caution about the difficulties and level of commitment, we offer some basic advice and recommend that readers consult experienced experts and books devoted to the subject.

Before creating a new project in a particular region or country, you should first learn the local language and culture, as well as the health problems and needs of that community. Knowing the national health priorities, the goals of the country's Ministry of Health, and the efforts of the various organizations in a region would also be extremely valuable. Involving government officials and local health workers at an early stage is important for receiving approval to initiate and conduct a project. Any project will need to include a local identification of needs and ownership. Addressing effective partnerships and identifying the issue of sustainability from the start of the project will also be important considerations. Having secure financial resources over a period of time is important, because stopping and starting projects may lead to significant frustration and mistrust from the communities. Finally, one should try to speak with other people who have set up their own health-related projects in developing countries, as they often will have valuable wisdom and advice to share.

Bringing Global Health Work Home

The problems of global health extend into issues within our 'home' communities, and some of the best 'global' health experiences do not require any travel abroad. In the inner cities of North America, there are scores of homeless people, injection drug users, and marginalized people infected with HIV or other sexually transmitted pathogens. The problems of poverty, poor access to health care services, and gender and racial stigma abound. The issues that we attempt to address as 'global health' issues in faraway resource-poor countries often need to be addressed within our own cities.

Problems of alcoholism, drug abuse, poor housing, suicide, and violence can be seen in many Aboriginal communities. Life expectancies can often be 20 years less in these Aboriginal communities compared with their non-Aboriginal counterparts. Aboriginal communities often have poor access to resources, financial support, and health care institutions to tackle many of their health problems. Their problems, like those of the marginalized inner city populations, are similar to the typical problems encountered in resource-poor settings around the world.

Many health care professionals who work in developing countries often return to discover similar situations within their own country. The lessons learned while working abroad with few resources – including human, financial, and systemic supports – can be similar to lessons learned at home while working with poor or marginalized populations. Furthermore, the creativity required to maximize health outcomes abroad may be applied in resource-poor settings at home.

An important word of advice for those who are interested in working abroad is that you don't have to travel abroad to do great global health work. The problems at home are as international and important as those abroad, and often you'll be helping disadvantaged populations in your own communities.

Identifying Your Goals

Now that the basic landscape of global health opportunities has been described, you can now identify your goals in pursuing a global health experience. This begins with understanding your own potential. If you haven't travelled to a developing country, then you may not have thought much about your comfort level in these situations. Would you feel comfortable living in a rural area that does not have running water or electricity? If not, then you should consider locations that are more urban or with more developed infrastructures. Do you have a health condition that requires you to be close to a health care facility? If so, then consider a location that is not too far from a health care facility for your comfort level. Knowing your own limits and abilities is important as you start to identify your goals.

Identifying your goals before initiating the search for your global health experience will allow you not only to tailor your efforts and search to relevant opportunities, but also will help you obtain a more suitable and rewarding experience. The process of identifying your goals does not have to be a long soul-searching affair, and it can be achieved by completing the following four tasks:

1 Identify the type of experience you are seeking from among the six major areas of global health opportunities.
2 Determine the optimal duration of your experience.
3 Determine if you want your experience to be in a specific country or geographical region.
4 Consider any special needs or circumstances.

To elaborate on the first task, identifying the type of experience you are seeking in global health involves many considerations, and we list some of the questions that you may ask yourself in Table 3.2. These questions are designed to help you first identify which of the six broad areas of global health opportunities are most suited to your interests and goals. You should determine the types of situations you like to work in: rural or urban, individual or in groups. Then, you should decide whether you are looking for an educational opportunity or a working experience. If you are looking for a working experience, you will need to determine whether you are qualified for clinical work, teaching abroad, or advocacy work, or if you wish to conduct research. If you are not interested in any of these areas, then you are most likely

Table 3.2
Identify Your Goals: Type of Experience

Do you want to do health research?
Are you qualified to do clinical/hospital work?
Do you want a rural, urban, or peri-urban setting?
Do you want to work as an individual or in a group situation?
Do you want to learn more about global health or tropical medicine?
Do you want to concentrate on learning a language?
Do you want to do global health work?
Do you envision having another type of global health experience?
Would you like to establish a new global health project?

Table 3.3
Identify Your Goals: Duration of Experience

How much time can you reasonably allocate for your experience?
Do you want to retain your employment and use vacation days?
Are you limited to a short-term work vacation or clinical rotation?
Do you want an experience that is longer than 6 months?
Are you looking for a long-term position or assignment?
Are you hoping to start a career in global health?

---

searching for either a short-term or long-term working opportunity, and you will need to consider the optimal duration of your experience, which we discuss next.

After determining the type of global health experience you are seeking, the next task is to consider the optimal duration for your global health experience. As has been described, experiences can range from a couple of weeks to several years to a lifelong career. Table 3.3 lists some questions that you might ask yourself prior to getting involved in global health. One of the biggest factors is whether or not you wish to retain your present employment. If you do, then you will be limited to short-term opportunities. If you are changing employment or are in a transition period, then you are in a better position to search for a long-term opportunity. You should also consider the challenges of living abroad for a long-term assignment. These might include coping with being away from family and friends, the need for financial or other support, and the experiences of your family if they join you, as well as adjusting to strange or unfamiliar environments and different foods and levels of sanitation and the frustrations that come with learning and speaking a new language. Anticipating how you may handle these situations, which may also add to the excitement of working in a developing country, will serve you better in the long run. You may also want to give some thought to how much time would be necessary or appropriate to accomplish the goals you have identified.

The next step is to determine if you want your experience to be in a specific country or geographical region. Do you want to be close to family? If so, then flights within the western hemisphere are generally easier and cheaper than travelling across several time zones. Do you speak additional languages? Certain languages such as Arabic, Portuguese, and Swahili would be valuable in certain regions of Africa. Of course, knowledge of local, indigenous languages would be highly valued for specific positions in more rural settings. The country's level of safety and stability should also be taken into consideration. The U.S. State Department maintains current information on international travel and security, while issuing appropriate travel warnings (http://travel.state.gov/travel/). The Canadian Department of Foreign Affairs and International Trade (www.voyage.gc.ca) has good information for Canadian travellers.

In addition to identifying the type, optimal duration, and location of your global health experience, there are several special needs or circumstances that should be taken into account. Some key questions to ask yourself are listed in Table 3.4. First, your personal health, safety, and well-being are paramount and vital when travelling abroad. Without first taking care of yourself, you will hardly be in a position to help others. Especially, if you are a high-risk patient or require specific medical services, you should pay attention to the location of an assignment. Individuals with medical conditions, elderly individuals, and pregnant women should have a frank discussion with their physician, and be prepared to carry with them all of the appropriate medications and medical documentation. Deciding when one is fit for working in a developing country can often be difficult and personally biased, but it is important not to put yourself into a situation where the required medical services are not available. In addition, you should not put yourself into a dangerous situation or try to do work that is beyond your abilities or level of comfort. Rushing into a volatile scene not only will put you at increased danger, but also could make you part of the health care problem. This generally applies to doing disaster relief or refugee-related work – these services should not be attempted on your own, but instead should be coordinated with an established organization.

Table 3.4
Identify Your Goals: Special Considerations

Do you have any special medical needs or concerns?
Are you fit to work in a rural area that has limited health services?
How does your spouse/partner feel about living abroad?
How would your children handle living in a developing country?
Is anything preventing you from accepting a global health position?
Are you adaptable to living conditions that may be less desirable than at home?
How much of your own money are you willing to contribute to achieve your goals?

In addition to your own needs, if you have a spouse or partner and/ or children, then considering their interests and needs will be especially important. Although living abroad with your family can be extremely enriching and can enhance your relationships, the foreign nature of the environment can also make it an extremely difficult situation. Some difficulties include language and cultural differences, the stress of international travel, safety and health concerns, financial matters, the education of your children, and diminished communication with family and friends. You should agree as a couple on the global health work or project; otherwise some resentment could quickly boil to the surface. Children raised in a developing country will benefit from another language and culture; however, the problems of fitting into a new and very different environment may be difficult. Having children should not be a hindrance to doing global health work, since adequate and affordable child care and education can be found in almost all developing countries. In fact, many major cities in developing countries have North American–style schools that offer a very good education. Finally, concerning older children, it is important to have a discussion on a regular basis to gauge their concerns and fears about living abroad.

Summary

This chapter has presented the six major areas of global health opportunities and the types of experiences that can be obtained within each area. Any one of these avenues can be pursued to initiate an experience or launch a career in global health. The process starts with identifying your goals. By identifying your goals you will be better suited to obtain a global health experience that is tailored to your interests and abilities. Start by asking yourself about your personality and motivation; this can help you determine the type of experience you are seeking. Next, identify the duration of your desired experience, while realizing that all types of opportunities, ranging from a couple of weeks to an entire career, exist. Finally, once you have identified the type and duration of work you are seeking, address some special considerations, such as personal health and safety and spousal and family issues. Having cleared these hurdles, you can now use the following chapters to get started in efficiently exploring the many global health opportunities available to you.

4 Medical Electives, Research Opportunities, Medical Language Courses, Health Courses and Seminars, and Global Health Conferences

Opportunities to become more engaged in global health activities and learning are abundant. This chapter provides information that is tailored to people who want to either do clinical work, conduct research, or learn more about global health issues. Experiences gained from the opportunities examined in this chapter can also be beneficial for obtaining work with a governmental or non-governmental organization (Chapter 5) or for pursuing more significant educational opportunities (Chapter 6). The opportunities listed in this chapter contain relevant descriptions and contact information. This information has been either published online or supplied by the organizations. Therefore, these people or organizations should be receptive to inquiries, but as programs change, some information may no longer be accurate. The most up-to-date information should be obtained by directly contacting the individuals or organizations. Although the information contained in this chapter is broad and has been compiled over several years, during the course of our professional careers, it is certainly not a complete listing of the available opportunities.

In this chapter, we provide listing for 61 international medical electives, 93 sites for medical language courses, 22 global health courses and seminars, and 15 global health conferences. In particular, several organizations and websites listed below are continually updated and can serve as more current repositories for medical elective information. Additional information about particular organizations can also be found in Chapter 5.

International Medical Electives and Volunteer Opportunities

Websites for International Medical Electives

American Academy of Family Physicians
www.aafp.org/cgi-bin/ihcop.pl

American College of Physicians
www.acponline.org/college/international/?hp

American College of Surgeons, Operation Giving Back
www.operationgivingback.facs.org

American Medical Student Association
www.amsa/org/global/ih/

Global Medicine
www.globalmedicine.org

International Medical Volunteers Association
www.imva.org

Medical Electives in Multiple Locations

Carefree Foundation
5530 Wisconsin Avenue, Suite 914, Chevy Chase, MD 20815
E-mail: info@carefreefoundation.org
Website: www.carefreefoundation.org
Highlights: Third- or fourth-year medical students can rotate in developing countries for 2 to 3 weeks.

Child Family Health International (CFHI)
995 Market Street, Suite 1104, San Francisco, CA 94103
Website: www.cfhi.org
Highlights: CFHI places medical students in electives and medical language courses in Bolivia, India, Amazon Basin, Mexico, South Africa and other countries.

International Federation of Medical Students Association–USA
(IFMSA–USA)
PO Box 1990, Philadelphia, PA 19105-1990
Website: www.ifmsa.org
Highlights: IFMSA–USA operates through the IFMSA–USA National

Exchange Officer (NEO) to coordinate the international exchange program. Clerkships of all types of specialties may be in nearly any country around the world. A participant must be a member of IFMSA–USA to participate.

Lalmba
Website: www.lalmba.org
Highlights: Lalmba has one clinic in Chiri, southwestern Ethiopia, and a second clinic in Matoso, adjacent to Lake Victoria. Living arrangements are not luxurious, but are quite comfortable and private. There are two to five volunteers at a site at any given time. Assignments are generally for 1 to 2 years. These sites are not for students.

Vanter Cruise Health Services (VCHS)
635 Slaters Lane, Suite 140, Alexandria, VA 22314
Website: www.vanterventures.com
Highlights: The Yale Emergency Medicine Residency in cooperation with VCHS offers a 4-week elective in cruise medicine to senior residents in emergency medicine. Physicians treat passengers and crew on the Disney Cruise Line.

CENTRAL AMERICA/CARIBBEAN

Barbados
Queen Elizabeth Hospital
Faculty of Medical Sciences, Bridgetown, Barbados
Phone: (246) 429-5112 or *Fax:* (246) 429-6738
Website: www.medicstravel.co.uk/Medics_Guide_To_Work_and_
Electives_Around_The_World/updates.htm
Highlights: The clerkship is held at the Queen Elizabeth Hospital in Bridgetown for most medical disciplines, except in family medicine and community health. The clerkship in family medicine is held at the General Practice Unit at the Edgar Cochrane Polyclinic, and the clerkship in community health is conducted at the Randal Phillips Polyclinic. Clinical electives will normally be 8 to 10 weeks. The University of the West Indies does not provide facilities for accommodation of elective students, but there are private lodgings available.

Belize
Hillside Healthcare Center

Hillside Health Care International, PO Box 151, Brookfield, WI 53008-0151
Phone: (608) 751-7672
Website: www.hillsidebelize.org
Highlights: This rotation is for medical/health students and medical residents from primary care specialties. A 4-week minimum commitment is requested.

Dominican Republic
Batey Relief Alliance
PO Box 300565, Brooklyn, NY 11230-5656
Website: www.bateyrelief.org
Highlights: The Batey Relief Alliance offers health and development programs for economically disadvantaged children and their families in the Caribbean. Opportunities for short-term volunteers are available for health professionals and students.

Village Mountain Mission (VMM)
Phone: (740) 603-3260
Website: www.oucom.ohiou.edu/international/VMM
Highlights: The Medical Mission Clinic in Luperon, Dominican Republic, combined with the Ohio University College of Osteopathic Medicine, visits for 10 days in early July to help provide medical screening, education support, and treat medical diseases and conditions.

El Salvador
Center for the Complete Development of Children and Their Families (CEDEINFA)
Ohio University, College of Osteopathic Medicine, Irvine Hall, Athens, OH 45701
Website: www.oucom.ohiou.edu/international
Highlights: Medical students work with inner city clinics and village 'brigades' to support the ongoing work of CEDEINFA to rescue high-risk children who live in the poorest communities of San Salvador.

Guatemala
SALUD
Res. Las Jacarandas #8-E, Antigua, Guatemala, Sacatepequez
Website: www.mundo-guatemala.com

Highlights: The SALUD programs of the International Health Elective by Mundo Guatemala are open to everybody working and/or studying in the area of medicine and health. Participants learn the language, culture, and traditions of Guatemala. Programs may include 20 hours per week private Spanish instruction, depending on existing language skills. Activities include visits to social projects, hospitals, public health and other health-related institutions, including weekend trips.

Haiti
Hôpital Albert Schweitzer
PO Box 81046, Pittsburgh, PA 15217
Phone: (412) 361-5200
Website: www.hashaiti.org/C2a.html
Highlights: Hôpital Albert Schweitzer has been helping the poor in Haiti for over 50 years. Many volunteer opportunities exist, and the hospital has continually accepted medical students on clinical elective rotations.

Honduras
Friends of Honduran Children
Website: www.honduranchildren.com
Highlights: Friends of Honduran Children send three Brigades a year consisting of 16 to 18 medical professionals who run several day clinics that provide medical and dental care to remote areas of Honduras.

Shoulder to Shoulder, Inc.
4754 Chapel Ridge Drive, Cincinnati, OH 45223
Website: www.shouldertoshoulder.org
Highlights: Shoulder to Shoulder seeks to address the health, economic, and education needs of the poorest areas of Honduras. Volunteer opportunities are available for medical residents and students.

Surgical Team, Developing World Medicine
Ohio University, College of Osteopathic Medicine, Irvine Hall, Athens, OH 45701
Website: www.oucom.ohiou.edu/international
Highlights: The 2-week trip consists of a week of 'surgical brigade' and a week of follow-up care of surgical patients, in addition to visits to health care facilities and a medical school.

SOUTH AMERICA

Argentina
Universidad del Salvador, School of Medicine
International Cooperation and Exchange Department
Rodríguez Peña 770 – Piso 1, (C1020ADP) Buenos Aires, Argentina
Website: www.salvador.edu.ar/medicina (English version)
Highlights: The main objective is to support all international educational opportunities for university students who want to complement their studies with an academic and cultural experience in a foreign country.

Ecuador
Clinical Rotation in Ecuador
Ohio University, College of Osteopathic Medicine, Irvine Hall, Athens, OH 45701
Website: www.oucom.ohiou.edu/international
Highlights: 4-week programs in selected hospitals in Ecuador include medical Spanish and rotations in different services offered by the participating hospitals.

Community-Based Tropical Disease Research in Ecuador
Ohio University, College of Osteopathic Medicine, Irvine Hall, Athens, OH 45701
Website: www.oucom.ohiou.edu/international
Highlights: Activities include a continuation of a Pilot Chagas Control project; 4-week minimum required.

Tropical Disease Biology Workshop
Ohio University, College of Osteopathic Medicine, Irvine Hall, Athens, OH 45701
Website: www.oucom.ohiou.edu/international
Highlights: The objective of this multidisciplinary adventure and field research experience is to gain a deeper understanding of the complex factors that play a role in the biology of tropical diseases.

Mondaña Medical Clinic (MMC) – Yachana Foundation
PO Box 17-17-185, Quito, Ecuador
Phone: (593 2) 223-7278/223-7133/222-2584

Website: www.yachana.org.ec/
Highlights: The MMC – Yachana Foundation (formerly FUNEDESIN) clinical rotation program is for medical students who want to experience the challenges of health care delivery in remote areas of Ecuador.

EUROPE

France
University of Marseilles
Website: www.timone.univ-mrs.fr/medecine/ri/crelations_english. html
Highlights: Students can choose a clinical rotation or research laboratory available to Marseilles students. There is an expectation that an exchange will occur with the host institution.

Ireland
Royal College of Surgeons in Ireland (RCSI)
123 St Stephens Green, Dublin 2, Ireland
Website: www.rcsi.ie
Highlights: Clinical electives of all subspecialties are available for 4 to 8 weeks at various hospitals. The RCSI will assist in finding appropriate housing.

Malta
Malta Medical School
Malta Medical Students Association – Electives Coordinator, Guardamangia Hill, Guardamangia, Malta MSD 09
Website: www.mmsa.org.mt/
Highlights: The Malta Medical School offers visiting medical students an elective clerkship in any specialty. They will assist in finding appropriate housing.

Scotland
University of Glasgow
Incoming Elective Enquiries, Wolfson Medical School Building, University Avenue, Glasgow, Scotland G12 8QQ
Website: www.gla.ac.uk/faculties/medicine/overseas.html
Highlights: Clinical electives of all specialties offered to medical students in their final year. Electives last a maximum of 6 weeks.

Sweden
Linköping University
Website: www.liu.se/education/exchange/health/health
Highlights: Staff members at the hospitals and other care institutions speak English, as do many patients. However, as English is not the native language, the situation may limit opportunities to have close patient interactions.

United Kingdom
Barts and the London, Queen Mary's School of Medicine and Dentistry
Student Office, Barts and the London SMD, Old Medical College Building, London E1 2AD, United Kingdom
Website: www.smd.qmul.ac.uk/undergraduate/electives/index.html
Highlights: Visiting students can do up to an 8-week rotation in any of the various specialties and subspecialties listed in the information package found at the website.

AFRICA

Kenya
Chogoria Hospital, PCEA Chogoria Hospital
PO Box 35, Chogoria, Kenya
E-mail: chogoria@africaonline.co.ke
Highlights: Chogoria Hospital is a Presbyterian mission hospital in rural Kenya on the slopes of Mt Kenya. Clinical electives require a minimum 2-month commitment for students or residents, and typically fill the positions up to a year in advance.

Kenyan Grandparents Study
Ohio University, College of Osteopathic Medicine, Irvine Hall, Athens, OH 45701
Website: www.oucom.ohiou.edu/international
Highlights: This research project takes place in a rural area in western Kenya and seeks to examine the impact of caregiving for orphaned children on the health and well-being of Luo elders.

Moi University
Administrative Officer, International Programmes Office, Moi University, PO Box 3900, Eldoret, Kenya
Phone: 254-053-43620

Website: www.mu.ac.ke/ipo/
Highlights: Moi University offers clinical electives from 1 to 6 weeks in duration.

SHARE Kenya–Ohio
Ohio University, College of Osteopathic Medicine, Irvine Hall, Athens, OH 45701
Website: www.oucom.ohiou.edu/international
Highlights: Fourth-year medical students will participate in direct patient care in this clinical program that delivers health care to rural western Kenya.

Tumutumu Hospital
PCEA Tumutumu Hospital, Private Bag, Karatina, Kenya
E-mail: tumutumuhospital@yahoo.com
Highlights: Tumutumu is a Presbyterian mission hospital in rural Kenya. It offers an excellent medical and surgical experience, and typically fills the positions up to a year in advance.

Malawi
Embangweni Hospital
PO Box 7, Embangweni, Mzimba District, Malawi
Website: embangweni.com/hospital.htm
Highlights: Embangweni Hospital is located in rural western Malawi, and requires a 2-month commitment from students or residents. It is a small, rural, Western-style hospital.

South Africa
University of Witwatersrand
Elective Office, Faculty of Health Sciences, 7 York Road, Parktown 2193, South Africa
Phone: 27-11-717-2025
Website: web.wits.ac.za/Academic/Health/Students/elective/
Highlights: The university offers clinical electives in a variety of specialties.

Tanzania
Kilimanjaro Christian Medical Centre (KCMC)
PO Box 3010, Moshi, Tanzania
Website: www.kcmc.ac.tz

Highlights: KCMC offers an excellent clinical elective, and has become known as one of the most prominent teaching hospitals in East Africa.

Physician Training Partnership (PTP)
Website: www.ptpafrica.org
Highlights: PTP advances specialized care in developing nations through a focused, collaborative training program in partner nations. Volunteer opportunities are available for neurosurgical residents, medical students, and other medical professionals who have completed their training.

Selian Lutheran Hospital
PO Box 3164, Arusha, Tanzania
Website: selianlh.habari.co.tz/
Highlights: Selian Lutheran Hospital is a 125-bed hospital in northern Tanzania affiliated with Kilimanjaro Christian Medical Center and Tumaini University. The minimum externship is 8 weeks and the minimum residency rotation is 4 weeks.

Shirati Health, Education and Development (SHED) Foundation
University of Southern California (USC), School of Medicine
Website: www.shedfoundation.org
Highlights: The work of the SHED Foundation is focused on the areas of health, education, and development in underserved Tanzania communities. The 3- to 6-week program offered by USC under the auspices of the foundation may include clinic and public health work.

ASIA

Cambodia
Angkor Hospital for Children – Friends without a Border
Angkor Hospital for Children, PO Box 50, Siem Reap, Cambodia
Friends without a Border, 1123 Broadway, Suite 1210, New York, NY 10010
Website: www.angkorhospital.org
Highlights: Visiting medical students may rotate on the inpatient, outpatient, or emergency department, or visit community-based projects, such as home care, mobile clinics, health centres, and village health volunteer projects. Hospital policy stipulates that medical students have observer status only. There are many opportunities to develop clinical

diagnostic skills as patients present with a range and degree of pathology often far more advanced than that seen in a developed country. Accommodations are usually available at the hospital house.

China
Hangzhou, China
Stanford University's Center for Education in Family and Community Medicine
Phone: (415) 904-8033
Website: www.viaprograms.org
Highlights: Program with Stanford University to study traditional Chinese medicine through lectures, hands-on-demonstration, and hospital rounds, for 4 weeks. The program partners with Chinese medical students.

Shanghai Medical University (SMU)
Foreign Students Office, 138 Yi Xue Yuan Road, Shanghai, China
Website: www.shmu.edu.cn/esmu.htm
Highlights: SMU offers short-term classes to learn Chinese, traditional Chinese medicine, including acupuncture, and culture for students or professionals. The training specialty, time, and duration can be discussed directly with SMU. Classes are set up with suitable teaching materials and various teaching methods, according to the different skills and interests of the applicants. An acupuncture class aims to introduce Chinese acupuncture therapy, and practical training is included. Students can learn Chinese in the morning and acupuncture in the afternoon.

Tibetan Traditional Medical College
Website: familymed.stanford.edu/Tibet
Highlights: Stanford University offers a clinical program to see patients with experienced preceptors while learning the basic theories of traditional Tibetan medicine in a seminar setting, and to learn about the public health situation in rural Tibet, as well as the Chinese national health care system. The program includes a 4-week rotation at the Tibetan Traditional Medical College and its affiliate hospital in Lhasa, Tibet. Seminars introduce traditional Tibetan medicine (history, theory, diagnosis, treatment), and there is an optional language training component in conversational Chinese or Tibetan. Students will have opportunities to take trips outside of Lhasa to visit other affiliate hospitals

and clinics. There will be English interpretation during all elective-related educational activities. Upon successful completion of the rotation, six quarter units of academic credit can be awarded from Stanford Medical School.

India
India Study Abroad Center (ISAC)
B1202 Meera Society, New Link Road,
Oshiwara, Jogeshwari, (West), Mumbai 400 102, India
Phone: (415) 287-0144
Website: www.indiastudyabroad.org
Highlights: Comprehensive programs for health care volunteers are offered in the areas of rural and public health, traditional medicine, HIV/AIDS, and Mumbai clinical rotations.

Comprehensive Rural Health Project, Jamkhed International Foundation
PO Box 291, Carrboro, NC 27510
PO Jamkhed, Dist. Ahmednagar 413 201, Maharashtra, India
Website: www.jamkhed.org
Highlights: Jamkhed International Foundation provides 1-month clinical and public health rotations and a 1-month community-based health and development course in Maharashtra, India.

Mediciti Institute of Medical Sciences (MIMS)
Ghanpur, RR District, AP, India
Website: mediciti.org
Highlights: The MIMS rotation goal is to provide a perspective of medical care in a rural and resource-limited setting.

AVSAR
Website: www.avsarindia.org/new/Volunteer.htm
Highlights: Public health, dental public health, and research electives in Mumbai are available. Students will be expected to work in a service-oriented experience for 6 to 7 days per week.

Vellore Christian Medical College (VCMC)
Vellore 632 002, India
Website: www.vellorecmc.org/student.htm

Highlights: VCMC offers many clinical rotations of 1 to 3 months in various specialties to medical students.

Israel

The Hebrew University of Jerusalem, School of Medicine
Jerusalem Society of Medical Students, PO Box 12272, Jerusalem 91120, Israel
Website: wzo.org.il/en/programs/
Highlights: Clinical clerkships are available in a variety of areas at the Hadassah University Hospital. Hebrew is required for some specialties.

Tel Aviv University
Electives Program, Sackler Faculty of Medicine, Tel Aviv 69978, Israel
Website: www.med.tau.ac.il/medicine/Electives
Highlights: Electives are available in a variety of areas, minimum of 3 weeks in length. Apply 4 to 8 months in advance.

Ben-Gurion University of the Negev
Public Relations Office, Faculty of Health Sciences, PO Box 653, Beer Sheva, 84105, Israel
Website: cmsprod.bgu.ac.il/eng/fohs
Highlights: Electives are available in most disciplines, and clinics are conducted at the Soroka University Medical Center in Beer Sheva, in local urban and rural primary medicine. Knowledge of Hebrew is preferred for certain departments.

Nepal

Himalayan Health Exchange
PO Box 610, Decatur, GA 30031-0610
Phone: (404) 929-9399
Website: www.himalayanhealth.com/about.htm
Highlights: Himalayan Health Exchange offers trips for students and health care professionals that typically last 14–19 days, but can be extended for up to 4 to 5 weeks.

Kathmandu Medical College – Teaching Hospital
Mr Bijay Sharma, Personnel Department
Website: www.kmc.edu.np
Highlights: The fee is 25 per week, and visiting students need to arrange

visa, travel, lodging, and food. They will assist in arranging appropriate housing.

Nepal Medical College (NMC) and Teaching Hospital
Attarkhel, Jorpati, Kathmandu, Nepal
Website: www.nmcth.edu/elective_program.php
Highlights: NMC is affiliated with Kathmandu University. Minimum 4-week electives are available in a variety of disciplines.

Patan Academy of Health Sciences
PAHS Office, Patan Hospital, PO Box 252, Kathmandu, Nepal
Website: www.pahs.edu.np
Highlights: Seeks volunteers for basic science instructors and clinical physicians with credentials and interests to teach medical students. Volunteer faculty are welcome to come for as little as 6 weeks.

Sri Lanka
University of Ruhuna
Assistant Registrar, Faculty of Medicine, PO Box 70, Galle, Sri Lanka
Website: www.ruh.ac.lk/Uni/medicine/Elective.html
Highlights: Applications for elective appointments in any discipline within the Faculty of Medicine, University of Ruhuna, and the specialties available in the Teaching Hospital, Galle, are considered.

Thailand
Chiang Mai University
Faculty of Medicine, 110 Intavaroros Ampur Muang, Chiang Mai 50200, Thailand
Website: www.med.cmu.ac.th/HOME/
Highlights: Chiang Mai University offers clinical rotations in a variety of medicine specialties.

OCEANIA

Australia
University of Sydney
Website: www.medfac.usyd.edu.au/futurestudent/electives/index.php
Highlights: Placements are up to 8 weeks in duration and may be clinical or research-based. Apply at least 9 months in advance.

University of Tasmania
Electives Coordinator, School of Medicine,
Private Bag 68, Hobart, Tasmania 7001, Australia
Website: www.healthsci.utas.edu.au/medicine/electives/index.html
Highlights: Medical students must be in their final year of medical school
at the time of the elective. Clinical elective placements are available
within the University of Tasmania's three teaching hospitals for a min-
imum of 4 weeks and a maximum period of 16 weeks in one specialty.

New Zealand
The University of Auckland
Teresa Timo, Student Administrative Assistant, Medical Programme
Directorate, Faculty of Medical and Health Sciences, Private Bag 92019,
85 Park Road, Grafton, Auckland, New Zealand
Website: www.health.auckland.ac.nz
Highlights: Clinical electives are available for all types of medical sub-
specialties for up to 10 weeks, February through November.

International Research Opportunities

Academic institutions, particularly in the United States, conduct much
of the research in global health and medicine. Therefore, research positions in global health can be found with ongoing projects being conducted by universities. Opportunities are available to applicants with
any level of training, from undergraduate students to doctoral graduates. In addition, global health research encompasses a wide array of
academic disciplines, including economics, anthropology, public health
services, epidemiology, and clinical medicine. Currently, there is a concentration of American universities conducting global health research.
However, as global health research continues to expand, researchers
and institutions will become more numerous and diverse.

Global health research positions are often not considered to be regular programs or opportunities. While some positions may be listed on
public sites, they can be difficult to find. Therefore, recent graduates
may need to be proactive in finding a research position in global health,
particularly the candidates with limited experience or training. The
first step in this process is determining what type of research position
you might be seeking. With that perspective, it would be easier to determine which universities or individual professors are conducting
research in your particular area of interest. Currently, much, but cer-

tainly not all, of the global health research is being conducted on HIV/AIDS, tuberculosis, and malaria. But, as the global health landscape changes, the focus of global health research will also evolve.

Current students should first inquire with relevant departments and professors within their home university. If global health research opportunities are not readily available, speaking with professors can lead to contacts with their colleagues who are conducting research in your field of interest. Conducting research in a resource-poor setting often takes some considerable time and effort. The time available during a summer may not be adequate to initiate or complete a research project. Focusing a thesis or dissertation project on a global health topic might be necessary in order to have adequate time to conduct the research. Any time constriction or restraints should be discussed with a research mentor before embarking on the project.

There are several funding opportunities that could support undergraduate and graduate students to conduct global health research. For recent university graduates, the Fulbright Scholarship, MacArthur Scholarship, and Rotary Scholarship all provide funding for 1 year of work in a foreign country, and can be used for global health research. One fellowship, the Fogarty/Ellison Clinical Research Fellowship, funded by the U.S. National Institutes of Health Fogarty International Center (FIC) and the Ellison Medical Foundation, supports graduate health science students to conduct a year of clinical research in a developing country. The FIC's International Research Scientist Development Award is designed to support U.S. post-doctoral scientists, who are committed to a career in international health research, conducting basic, behavioural, or clinical research. More information about scholarships and fellowships that support global health research is available in Chapter 7.

Currently, much of the health research being conducted by universities in developing countries is funded through the FIC. Below, we present a listing of the FIC's major grants and the recipient institutions. Detailed contact information about the principal investigators and location of each research project can be obtained at the Fogarty International Center's website (www.fic.nih.gov). Health researchers working in a particular field can also be located through the National Library of Medicine's PubMed listing of publications (www.pubmed.gov). Either way, researchers are aware that their information is publicly available, and most are used to addressing inquiries about their projects and employment opportunities.

Certainly not all global health research comes from FIC grants, and several Canadian organizations also fund global health research. The Canadian Institutes of Health Research (www.cihr-irsc.gc.ca) is the national funding agency that supports research efforts in global health–related fields. In addition, the Global Health Research Initiative (www.ghri.ca) was recently formed as a partnership between four agencies to enhance Canada's global health research. These agencies are expected to increase opportunities in global health research over the coming years.

FIC's AIDS International Training and Research Program (AITRP) supports HIV/AIDS-related research training to strengthen the capacity of institutions in low- and middle-income countries. Currently funded programs include:

- Albert Einstein College of Medicine of Yeshiva University
- Baylor College of Medicine
- Brown University, Miriam Hospital
- Case Western Reserve University, School of Medicine
- Columbia University, Mailman School of Public Health
- Cornell University, Weill Medical College
- Dartmouth Medical School, Dartmouth–Hitchcock Medical Center
- Duke University, Medical Center
- Emory University, School of Medicine
- Harvard University, School of Public Health
- Johns Hopkins University, Bloomberg School of Public Health
- Mount Sinai School of Medicine, Division of Infectious Diseases
- New York University, School of Medicine
- Northwestern University, Feinberg School of Medicine
- State University of New York, Downstate Medical Center
- University of California, Berkeley, School of Public Health
- University of California, Los Angeles, School of Public Health
- University of Illinois at Chicago, School of Public Health
- University of Maryland at Baltimore, School of Medicine
- University of Miami, School of Medicine
- University of Nebraska at Lincoln, Nebraska Center for Virology
- University of North Carolina at Chapel Hill, Division of Infectious Diseases
- University of Pittsburgh, Graduate School of Public Health
- University of South Florida, College of Medicine

- University of Washington, Harborview Medical Center
- Vanderbilt University Medical Center, Institute for Global Health
- Yale University, School of Medicine

FIC's International Training and Research Program in Environmental and Occupational Health supports research training in general environmental health and occupational health. Currently funded programs include:

- California Department of Health Services, Environmental Health Investigations Branch
- Columbia University, Mailman School of Public Health
- Emory University, Rollins School of Public Health
- Michigan State University, Institute of International Health
- Mount Sinai School of Medicine, Division of Environmental and Occupational Medicine
- University of Alabama at Birmingham
- University of California, Berkeley, School of Public Health
- University of California, Davis, Pulmonary and Critical Care Medicine
- University of California, Los Angeles, Center for Occupational and Environmental Health
- University of Illinois at Chicago, Great Lakes Center for Occupational Environmental Safety and Health
- University of Iowa, Center for International Rural and Environmental Health
- University of Medicine and Dentistry of New Jersey, Environmental and Occupational Health
- University of Michigan, Department of Environmental Health Sciences
- University of Texas, Health Sciences Center at Houston, SW Center for Occupational Health
- University of Washington, Occupational and Environmental Medicine
- Yale University, School of Medicine

FIC's Global Infectious Disease Research Training Program (GID) supports research training needs related to infectious diseases that are predominantly endemic in or have an impact upon people living in developing countries. Currently funded programs include:

- Aga Khan University, Pakistan
- Baylor College of Medicine
- Case Western Reserve University
- Christian Medical College, India
- Cornell University
- Emory University
- Federal University of Bahia
- Harvard School of Public Health
- Johns Hopkins School of Public Health
- Massachusetts General Hospital
- National Institute of Public Health
- New York State Department of Health
- New York University
- Pennsylvania State University
- Seattle Biomedical Research Institution
- Southwest Foundation for Biomedical Research
- U.S. Naval Medical Research Center
- Universidad Peruana Cayetano Heredia, Peru
- University of California, Berkeley
- University of California, Davis
- University of California, Irvine
- University of California, San Diego
- University of California, San Francisco
- University of Cape Town, South Africa
- University of Georgia
- University of Maryland
- University of New Mexico
- University of North Carolina
- University of Pittsburgh
- University of Texas Medical Branch
- University of Virginia
- Yale University
- Yeshiva University

FIC's International Clinical, Operational, and Health Services Research and Training Award (ICOHRTA) for non-communicable diseases and disorders supports training to facilitate collaborative, multidisciplinary, international clinical, operational, health services and prevention science research between U.S. institutions and those in low-to middle-income countries. Currently funded programs include:

- Children's Hospital Boston, Department of Medicine
- Harvard University Medical School, Department of Social Medicine
- Michigan State University, Department of Epidemiology
- Tulane University, School of Public Health and Tropical Medicine
- University of Alabama at Birmingham, Division of Preventive Medicine
- University of California, Berkeley, School of Public Health
- University of California, Davis, College of Agriculture and Environmental Sciences
- University of California, Los Angeles, School of Public Health
- University of California, San Francisco, Epidemiology and Biostatistics
- University of Michigan, Department of Psychiatry
- University of North Carolina, Chapel Hill, Department of Social Medicine
- University of Rochester Medical Center, Department of Psychiatry
- Vanderbilt University, Peabody College
- Washington University, Department of Psychiatry

FIC's International Maternal and Child Health Research Training Program (MCH) supports building research capacity on maternal and child health issues in low- and middle-income countries. Currently funded programs include:

- Cornell University, Division of Nutritional Sciences
- Georgetown University, Department of Biology
- Harvard University, School of Public Health
- Tufts University, School of Medicine
- Tulane University, School of Public Health and Tropical Medicine
- University of Alabama at Birmingham, School of Medicine
- University of California, Davis, Department of Nutrition
- University of Iowa, Department of Pediatrics
- University of Miami, Department of Pediatrics
- University of Michigan, School of Public Health
- University of Pennsylvania, School of Medicine

FIC's International Training and Research Program in Population and Health (POP) supports research training in population-related sciences. Currently funded programs include:

- Johns Hopkins University
- Oregon Health Sciences University
- University of California, Berkeley
- University of California, Los Angeles
- University of Colorado, Boulder
- University of Michigan
- University of North Carolina, Chapel Hill
- University of Virginia
- University of Wisconsin
- Virginia Commonwealth University

FIC's International Clinical, Operational, and Health Services Research and Training Award (ICOHRTA) for AIDS/TB supports research training where AIDS, TB, or both are significant problems. Currently funded programs include:

- Case Western Reserve University
- Cornell University, Weill Medical College
- Johns Hopkins University
- Stanford University
- University of California, Los Angeles
- Yale University

FIC's International Collaborative Genetics Research Training Program supports promoting equitable international collaborations for the advancement of sustainable genetic science. Currently funded programs include:

- Columbia University, Genome Center
- Johns Hopkins University, Institute of Genetic Medicine
- University of Pittsburg, Human Genetics Department
- University of Texas Health Science Center at San Antonio, Department of Psychiatry
- University of Pittsburgh Medical Center, Western Psychiatric Institute and Clinic
- Yale/VA Connecticut Health Care System, Department of Psychiatry

FIC's International Studies on Health and Economic Development (ISHED) supports research that examines the effects of health on macroeconomic performance of countries or on microeconomic agents utilizing longitudinal, comparative, and experimental forms of analysis. Currently funded programs include:

- Emory University
- Princeton University
- Rand Corporation
- University of North Carolina, Chapel Hill
- University of Pennsylvania

Here is a brief listing of other FIC grant programs that support global health research. The International Collaborative Trauma and Injury Research Training Program (ICTIRT) is a new grant that supports research on the growing burden of morbidity and mortality in the developing world due to trauma and injury. The Informatics Training for Global Health grant supports the development of informatics training programs. The Health, Environment, and Economic Development (HEED) Program is designed to research linkages between health, environment, and economic development. The Ecology of Infectious Diseases funds projects that strive to elucidate the underlying ecological and biological mechanisms that govern the relationships between environmental changes and the transmission dynamics of infectious diseases. Finally, the Brain Disorders in the Developing World: Research Across the Lifespan grant supports research relevant to brain disorders in low- and middle-income nations.

Medical Language Courses

Courses that combine foreign language study with a component of global health and medicine have been growing steadily since the 1980s. There are now numerous courses for various languages, but the vast majority of them are Spanish-language courses.

Inherent in the large number of offerings are large variations of the foreign language and global health combination. While most courses are rather balanced, some emphasize the language component, whereas others may stress the global health component. Furthermore, within the language and global health components lies much variety. Language study may be in the form of individual instruction or group classes of a small to large size. Classes may be offered for a few hours a day or for the entire day, and the classrooms may or may not be well equipped, quiet, and private. Some courses may expect or require a certain degreè of prior language knowledge or fluency. The inclusion of medical terminology and phrases will also vary from one course to another. Similarly, any global health portion of a course may be comprised of some hands-on medical work, health lectures, tours of clinics, and or observation of health care workers. The cost of medical language courses will vary considerably, and is typically based on content, location, and amenities provided, such as transportation, housing, and food. Therefore, individuals who have an interest in language study merged with global health are advised to compare the options, noting the various models being offered.

Although it is difficult to know about the quality of the course or location before attending, it may be worthwhile to contact previous participants of a course. Most programs are willing to provide this information to potential applicants, and past participants often give honest, candid advice about a program. A program's website will provide some valuable information and the Internet is a good starting place for comparing medical language courses. Below, we note the websites for 86 different medical Spanish language courses in locations throughout Latin America and Spain, as well as seven medical language (French, German, and Italian) courses located elsewhere. *Only courses for which a detailed description or syllabus was provided are included in this list.*

LATIN AMERICA/SPAIN

Argentina
Latin Immersion Language Network
www.latinimmersion.com

SALUD
www.amerispan.com/salud

Verbum School of Spanish
www.verbum.biz

Bolivia
Academia Latinoamericana de Español
www.latinoschools.com

Child Family Health International
www.cfhi.org

National Registration Center for Study Abroad
www.ncrsa.com

Chile
Adelante, LLC
www.adelanteabroad.com

Latin Immersion Language Network
www.latinimmersion.com

SALUD
www.amerispan.com/salud

Costa Rica
Adventure Education Center
www.adventurespanishschool.com

Centro Panamericano de Idiomas
www.spanishlanguageschool.com

International Health Central America Institute
www.ihcai.org

Instituto de Cultura y Lengua Costarricense
www.iclc.ws

Instituto Profesional de Español para Extranjeros
www.ipee.com

Montana State University
www.montana.edu/international/studyabroad/summer_programs/
costa_rica.htm

National Registration Center for Study Abroad
www.ncrsa.com

Rancho de Español
www.ranchodeespanol.com

Spanish Abroad, Inc.
www.spanishabroad.com/prog_medical.htm

Universal de Idiomas
www.universal-edu.com

Dominican Republic
Hispaniola Spanish Language School
www.hispaniola.org/home.htm

Ecuador
Academia de Español Surpacifico
www.surpacifico.k12.ec

Academia Latinoamericana de Español
www.latinoschools.com

Cacha Medical Spanish Institute
www.cachamsi.com

Center for Interamerican Studies
www.cedei.org

Child Family Health International
www.cfhi.org

Interhealth South America
www.interhealthsouthamerica.net

National Registration Center for Study Abroad
www.ncrsa.com

SALUD
www.amerispan.com/salud

Guatemala
Asociación Pop-Wuj
www.pop-wuj.org

Casa de Lenguas
www.casadelenguas.com

Ixchel Spanish School
www.ixchelschool.com

Mayan Medical Aid
www.mayanmedicalaid.org

Miguel Angel Asturias Spanish School
www.spanishschool.com

Ohiyesa
john.h.lyons@dartmouth.edu

SALUD
www.amerispan.com/salud

SALUD in Guatemala
www.mundo-guatemala.com

Mexico
Academia Falcon AC
www.academiafalcon.com

Adelante, LLC
www.adelanteabroad.com

Baja California Language College
www.bajacal.com

Cancun Spanish Language Institute
www.studyspanish-mexico.com

Cemanahuac Educational Community
www.cemanahuac.com

Centro Bilingue
www.van-graff.com/cuernavaca/index2.html

Centro de Arte y Lenguas Ibero-Azteca
www.prodigyweb.net.mx/calia

Centro de Idiomas, Cultura, and Comunicación
www.cicclapaz.com

CETLALIC Alternative Language School
www.cetlalic.org.mx

Child Family Health International
www.cfhi.org

Cuernavaca Language School
www.cuernavacalanguageschool.com

Don Quijote
www.donquijote.org

English/Spanish for All
www.mexonline.com/efa.htm

Healthwrights Spanish Training Program
www.healthwrights.org

Instituto Chac-Mool
www.chac-mool.com

Instituto Cultural Oaxaca
www.instculturaloax.com.mx

Instituto de Comunicación y Cultura
www.iccoax.com

Instituto Mexico Americano de Cultura
www.spanish-school.com.mx

Interamerican Universities Studies Institute
www.iusi.org/programs/workshops

International Community Health and Medical Spanish
www.medicalspanish.org

International House Riviera Maya
www.ihrivieramaya.com

Mar de Jade
www.mardejade.com

Medical Spanish Immersion
www.medicalspanish.homestead.com

MedSpanish
www.medspanish.com

National Registration Center for Study Abroad
www.ncrsa.com

Rios Associates
www.proespanol.com

SALUD
www.amerispan.com/salud

Se Habla ... La Paz
www.sehablalapaz.com

Spanish Abroad, Inc.
www.spanishabroad.com/prog_medical.htm

Universidad Autónoma de Guadalajara
www.uag.mx

Universidad Internacional
www.spanishschool.uninter.edu.mx

Nicaragua
¡Viva! Spanish School
www.vivaspanishschool.com

Panama
Spanish Abroad, Inc.
www.spanishabroad.com/prog_medical.htm

Peru
Academia Latinoamericana de Español
www.latinoschools.com

Amauta Spanish School
www.amautaspanish.com

National Registration Center for Study Abroad
www.ncrsa.com

Peru Language Center
www.perulanguage.com

Proyecto Peru
www.proyectoperucentre.org

SALUD
www.amerispan.com/salud

Wiracocha Spanish School
www.wiracochaschool.org

Spain
Babel Idiomas
www.babelidiomas.com

Elemadrid
www.elemadrid.com

Escuela Internacional
www.escuelai.com/spanish_course_medical_students.html

Linc School of Spanish
www.linc.tv

National Registration Center for Study Abroad
www.ncrsa.com

SALUD
www.amerispan.com/salud

Spanish Abroad, Inc.
www.spanishabroad.com/prog_medical.htm

Uruguay
Adelante, LLC
www.adelanteabroad.com

Venezuela
Centro de Linguistica Aplicada
www.cela-ve.com

Jakera Language School
www.learn-spanish-in-latin-america.com

OTHER

Canada
Medical French
http://www.collegecanada.com/aca_language.php

France
Àlliance Française
www.alliancefr.org/

Anglo French Medical Society (AFMS)
www.anglofrenchmedical.org

Medical French
www.bls-frenchcourses.com/

Germany
Medical German
http://www.studyabroadinternational.com/Germany/Hamburg/
Germany_Hamburg_courses.html

Italy
Course of Medical Italian
www.italianoespresso.com

Italian of Medicine and Science
www.porta-doriente.com/italian%20language%20school/italian_
science.htm

International Health Courses and Seminars

Courses and seminars provide excellent opportunities to learn more about global health or new areas of global health while networking with other people interested in global health and medicine. These courses are typically completed in several weeks to months and are less of a commitment than a typical 1- to 2-year master's degree program. In the following section, 22 of the most prominent and well-recognized courses are described. However, this listing is by no means comprehensive of all short courses and seminars available in global health. An additional general resource for global health courses can be found at www.health training.org. Some of the programs listed are for physicians or clinical practitioners who wish to become qualified in tropical medicine. Two certificate programs for physicians and clinical practitioners are well recognized. First, the American Society of Tropical Medicine and Hygiene offers a test for accreditation in tropical medicine and traveller's health. Second, several schools around the world offer a course leading to a diploma in tropical medicine and hygiene. Several other programs are for undergraduate students, and medical students, public health practitioners, as well as those with little experience. The programs are listed alphabetically by the sponsoring institution and use quotation marks when text is obtained directly from the organization. All of these courses and seminars, to our knowledge, are held on an annual basis.

'Diploma in Tropical Medicine and Hygiene,' London School of
Hygiene and Tropical Medicine
Description: Combines practical laboratory work, a series of lectures and seminars, and some clinical experience designed to provide doctors with the clinical and factual knowledge that will form the basis of professional competence in tropical medicine.
Location and Month: London, England, 3 months from January to March.

Target Participants: Recently qualified physicians to specialist infectious disease physicians.
Website: www.lshtm.ac.uk/prospectus/short/stmh.html

'International Honors Program on Health and Community,' Boston University
Description: Offers participants an opportunity to learn about the many factors that influence how individuals and groups respond to the health consequences of their genetic, environmental, and social circumstances. The course creates a framework for understanding systems that affect health on local, national, historic, and international levels.
Location and Month: Begins in Boston and includes visits to various countries, 4 months from January to May.
Target Participants: Undergraduate students interested in health care on a global scale.
Website: www.ihp.edu/programs/hc

'The Gorgas Course in Clinical Tropical Medicine,' Gorgas Memorial Institute and the University of Alabama at Birmingham
Description: Lectures, case conferences, diagnostic laboratory and daily bedside teaching in a 36-bed tropical medicine unit; taught in English.
Location and Month: Lima, Peru, 9 weeks from January to March.
Target Participants: Physicians, nursing professionals, physician assistants, and public health professionals.
Website: info.dom.uab.edu/

'Courses in Tropical Medicine,' Bernhard Nocht Institute for Tropical Medicine
Description: Doctors taking interests in infectious diseases and in the care of patients travelling or migrating from and to tropical and subtropical regions; taught in German.
Location and Month: Hamburg, Germany, in April.
Target Participants: Clinical practitioners, especially internal and general medicine physicians.
Website: www15.bmi-hamburg.de/bni/bni2/neu2/getfile.acgi?area_engl=courses&pid=510

'Summer Public Health Program,' Council on International Educational Exchange
Description: To teach students public health in underdeveloped setting; taught in Spanish.

Location and Month: Santiago, Dominican Republic, 7 weeks from May to July.
Target Participants: Students with an interest in Spanish language, medicine, and the allied health professions in the context of underdevelopment and public health.
Website: www.ciee.org/program_search/program_detail.aspx? program_id=125

'Program on Ethical Issues in International Health Research,' Harvard School of Public Health
Description: To discuss ethical issues related to international health work and research.
Location and Month: Boston, Massachusetts, 5 days in June.
Target Participants: International health researchers.
Website: www.hsph.harvard.edu/bioethics

'Summer Course on Refugee Issues,' York University's Centre for Refugee Studies
Description: Offers post-graduate training in refugee issues for practitioners who work on some aspect of refugee protection or assistance. The course includes panel discussions, case studies, a simulation exercise, and lectures from international experts.
Location and Month: Toronto, Canada, 8 days in June.
Target Participants: Academic and field-based practitioners working in the areas of forced migration.
Website: www.yorku.ca/crs/summer.htm

'Summer Institute in Reproductive Health and Development,' Johns Hopkins Bloomberg School of Public Health
Description: To strengthen training in reproductive health research and enhance leadership skills. The course uses a multidisciplinary approach to address reproductive health and development, combining contemporary issues in reproductive health, research methods, and leadership training. A limited number of scholarships may be available to individuals from developing countries.
Location and Month: Baltimore, Maryland, in June.
Target Participants: Mid-career professionals working in developing countries in population and reproductive health.
Website: www.jhsph.edu/GatesInstitute

'Graduate Summer Institute of Epidemiology and Biostatistics,' Johns Hopkins Bloomberg School of Public Health
Description: The program is intended to develop an understanding of basic and advanced principles of epidemiological research, and presents epidemiological methods and their application to the study of the natural history and etiology of disease.
Location and Month: Baltimore, Maryland, 4 weeks in June and July.
Target Participants: Provides an opportunity for graduate study to degree candidates as well as individuals taking selected courses for professional development.
Website: www.jhsph.edu/summerEpi

'Summer Institute in Tropical Medicine and Public Health,' Johns Hopkins Bloomberg School of Public Health
Description: To provide training in tropical medicine and related public health issues through a multidisciplinary approach, and to prepare participants for working with current and emerging health problems in developing countries and health problems of travellers. The course is designed as four 2-week modules.
Location and Month: Baltimore, Maryland, 8 weeks from June to August (can take any or all 2-week modules).
Target Participants: Physicians and other health care professionals.
Website: www.jhsph.edu/tropic

'Study Abroad Program in International Health,' Miami University
Description: Two courses ('International Health: A Global Perspective' and 'A European Perspective: Health, Social, Economic, and Political Impacts of Health Promotion') are taught, and students attend seminars at national and international organizations.
Location and Month: France and Switzerland, 5 weeks in June and July.
Target Participants: Undergraduate and graduate students.
Website: www.units.muohio.edu/eap/departments/phe/studyabroad.htm

'Tropical Disease Biology Workshop,' Tropical Disease Institute of Ohio University
Description: This is an observational and research program that takes place in Ecuador.
Location and Month: Ecuador, 2 weeks in June and July.

Target Participants: Undergraduate, graduate, medical, and non-degree students.
Website: www.oucom.ouiou.edu

'The HELP (Health Emergencies in Large Populations) Course,' International Committees of the Red Cross and Red Crescent Societies
Description: To upgrade professionalism in humanitarian assistance programs conducted in emergency situations.
Location and Month: Multiple locations around the world. Johns Hopkins University in July, 3 weeks.
Target Participants: Workers in complex humanitarian emergencies.
Website: www.jhsph.edu/Refugee/HELP/index.html

'China Public Health Summer Program Abroad for Public Health Students,' Tulane University's School of Public Health and Tropical Medicine
Description: Students will have the opportunity to learn about China's major health problems and take two courses: comparative health systems and health economics. These courses will be accompanied by first-hand visits to hospitals, private clinics, and health departments as well as guest lectures from local Chinese experts and health practitioners.
Location and Month: Shanghai, China, in July.
Target Participants: Students interested in the urban and rural health systems of China.
Website: www.sph.tulane.edu/hsm/pages/programs/phsummer.htm

'International Course in Tropical Medicine,' Louisiana State University Health Science Center and the University of Costa Rica Faculty of Medicine
Description: The course aims to provide students an insight into the impact of tropical diseases on the population of affected areas. It is a mixture of lectures, discussions, laboratory exercises, and some clinical presentations. Students do not participate in direct patient care. Teaching sites include the hilly southwest, the lowlands of the northeast and coastal east, and the high central plateau.
Location and Month: Costa Rica, in July.
Target Participants: Medical students, interns, residents or graduate students, and nurses working towards an advanced degree who have an interest in tropical medicine and parasitology.

Website: www.medschool.lsuhsc.edu/student_affairs/electives/
Microbiology.htm

'Basic Concepts in Global Health,' Universidad Peruana Cayetano
Heredia (UPCH)
Description: This course is a hands-on fast-paced immersion into the
complexities of global health. There are lectures, readings, informatics
training, and a research workshop.
Location and Month: Lima, Peru, in July.
Target Participants: Undergraduate students.
Website: www.globalhealthperu.org

'International Health in the Developing World,' University of Arizona.
Description: A multidisciplinary, case-based, problem-solving course
preparing medical students and primary care residents for health care
experiences in developing countries.
Location and Month: Tucson, Arizona, 3 weeks in July.
Target Participants: Medical students in years 3 and 4, primary care residents, or health professionals with clinical experience in any medical or
public health field.
Website: www.globalhealth.arizona.edu/IHIndex.html

'Annual Global Health Course,' University of Minnesota, Department
of Medicine
Description: This course will prepare attendees to work in global health,
including tropical medicine, traveller's health, and refugee and
migrant health.
Location and Month: Minneapolis, Minnesota, 8 weeks in July and
August.
Target Participants: Physicians and other health care providers working
in tropical medicine, traveller's health, and migrant health.
Website: www.globalhealth.umn.edu/globalhlth/course.html

'Diploma Course in Clinical Tropical Medicine and Travelers' Health,'
Tulane University, School of Public Health and Tropical Medicine
Description: To provide a structured curriculum with practical instruction in tropical medicine, including the pathophysiology, clinical fea-
tures, diagnosis, treatment, and control of diseases prevalent in the
tropics.

Location and Month: New Orleans, Louisiana, 4 months from August to December.
Target Participants: Physicians and other health professionals seeking certification in tropical medicine and traveller's health.
Website: www.sph.tulane.edu/tropmed/programs/diploma.htm

'Diploma in Tropical Medicine and Hygiene,' Liverpool School of Tropical Medicine
Description: The aim of the course is to equip physicians with the knowledge and skills needed to practise medicine and promote health in the tropics effectively.
Location and Month: Liverpool, England, 3 months, commencing September, May, or February.
Target Participants: Physicians who intend to or who are already practising in the tropics.
Website: www.liv.ac.uk/lstm/learning_teaching/post_grad/DiplTropMedHyg.htm

'Clinical Tropical Medicine and Parasitology Course,' West Virginia University
Description: The course focuses on the imparting of essential skills and competencies in clinical tropical medicine, laboratory skills in a low-technology setting, epidemiology and disease control, and traveller's health.
Location and Month: Morgantown, West Virginia, 8 weeks in the summer.
Target Participants: Health care professionals.
Website: www.hsc.wvu.edu/som/tropmed

'Epidemiology and Control of Infectious Diseases,' Imperial College London, Department of Infectious Disease Epidemiology
Description: This short course has 'demystified' mathematical modelling and kept public health researchers up to date with the fast-moving field, including pandemic influenza, SARS, HIV/AIDS, foot-and-mouth disease, and others.
Location and Month: London, England, in September.
Target Participants: Those interested in communicable disease tracking.
Website: www.imperial.ac.uk/cpd/epidemiology

'Global Health Leadership Institute,' American Medical Students Association

Description: To prepare medical students to be leaders in issues in global health and human rights.
Location and Month: Washington, DC, 3 days in September.
Target Participants: Medical students.
Website: www.amsa.org/global

Global Health Conferences

Several conferences related to or including global health topics are held around the world each year. Many conferences are devoted specifically to global health topics, while others related to public health may include global health issues. In this section, we present the most prominent conferences that address global health issues. We have attempted to present only conferences that are held on a regular basis, and not symposiums, summits, or one-time conferences. The following 15 conferences, presented in order by month of the conference, are among the most prominent conferences for global health and medicine.

National Convention of the International Federation of Medical Students Association – USA
Location and Month: Rotating in the United States, January
Target Participants: Medical students interested in global health

WONCA Rural Health Conference
Location and Month: Rotating around the world, February
Target Participants: Health professionals interested in health care among rural populations
Website: ruralwonca2008.net

Western Regional International Health Conference sponsored by the University of Washington, University of Arizona, and Oregon Health Sciences University
Location and Month: Rotating in the western United States, February
Target Participants: Students and professionals interested in global health
Website: depts.washington.edu/ihg

Annual Convention of the American Medical Students Association
Location and Month: Rotating in the United States, March or April
Target Participants: Medical students (includes global health topics)

Website: www.amsa.org/conv

Annual Global Health Education Consortium Conference
Location and Month: Rotating in North America and Central America,
April
Target Participants: Students, academics, and professionals interested in
global health
Website: www.globalhealth-ec.org

Unite for Sight Annual International Health Conference
Location and Month: Rotating in the United States, April
Target Participants: People interested in international service, global
health, public health, and medicine
Website: www.uniteforsight.org

Mount Sinai Global Health Conference
Location and Month: New York City, April
Target Participants: Medical students and professionals interested in
global health
Website: mssm-ghc.org

Annual Northern California International Health Conference sponsored by the Bay Area International Health Interest Group, University
of California at Davis, University of California at Berkeley, University
of California at San Francisco, Stanford University, and Kaiser Perma-
nente
Location and Month: Rotating in northern California, April
Target Participants: Students, researchers, and practitioners interested in
global health, medical and public health professionals, NGOs, community health workers, veterinarians, the media, policy makers at every
level, and the general public
Website: www.phs.ucdavis.edu/Intl/International.php

INMED Exploring Medical Missions Conference, sponsored by the
Institute for International Medicine
Location and Month: Kansas City, Missouri, May
Target Participants: Health practitioners and students interested in glo-
bal health service
Website: www.inmed.us/conference.asp

International Conference on Global Health of the Global Health Council
Location and Month: Washington, DC, May or June
Target Participants: Global health practitioners, researchers, advocates,
policy makers, and leaders
Website: www.globalhealth.org/conference

International AIDS Conference by the International AIDS Society
Location and Month: Rotates globally, August
Target Participants: Stakeholders involved in the global response to
HIV/AIDS
Website: www.iasociety.org

Canadian Conference on International Health by the Canadian Society
for International Health and the Canadian Coalition for Global Health
Research
Location and Month: Ottawa, Canada, October and November
Target Participants: Practitioners, researchers, educators, policy makers,
and community advocates
Website: www.csih.org/en/ccih/index.asp

Annual Meeting and Exposition of the American Public Health Association
Location and Month: Rotating in the United States, October and November
Target Participants: Public health professionals and students (includes
global health topics)
Website: www.apha.org/meetings

Annual Meeting of the American Society for Tropical Medicine and
Hygiene
Location and Month: Rotating in the United States, November
Target Participants: Scientists interested in tropical medicine and
hygiene
Website: www.astmh.org

Global Missions Health Conference by the Southeast Christian Church
Location and Month: Rotating in the United States, November
Target Participants: Students and professionals interested in global
health
Website: www.medicalmissions.com

5 Governmental and Non-Governmental Organizations

There are many types of organizations involved in coordinating and conducting global health work. Governmental organizations may either operate on behalf of several countries, such as the World Health Organization, or a single country, such as the Canadian International Development Agency. Non-governmental health organizations have more variety in their background, goals, and motivations. They may be private or public, for-profit or not-for-profit, and religiously affiliated or not religiously affiliated. In this chapter, the most prominent governmental and non-governmental organizations working in global health and medicine are presented and briefly described. Some organizations listed in this chapter, primarily foundations, may serve more as funding agencies for health projects, rather than implementers of health projects, in developing countries. Although this is a long list of organizations, it is by no means exhaustive. In addition, information about these organizations will change rapidly.

International Governmental Health Organizations

Many governmental organizations have been involved in global health and medicine work for a long time. Governmental organizations may be associated with a single government or may be composed of a body of representatives from several member countries. Although international government health agencies work to improve the health of people in other countries, they still operate under their national political and economic agendas. Most of the single-government agencies presented in this guidebook are based in the United States, Canada, or the United Kingdom, since other country governments may require native language speakers. The work of all governmental health organizations is typically influenced by the political climate, and can shift dramatically when new people or political parties enter office. In this section, we present most of the prominent governmental organizations that conduct health-related work in countries around the world. The list is presented alphabetically by the organization's name, followed by a brief description of what it does, the location of its headquarters, and the url for its website.

Canadian International Development Agency (CIDA)
Description: Canada's leading development agency, CICA works with partners around the world to support sustainable development in developing countries and to offer humanitarian assistance in areas of need. CIDA is increasingly placing its focus on a core group of 25 countries, most of which are in Africa.
Location: Hull, QC.
Website: www.acdi-cida.gc.ca

Centers for Disease Control and Prevention (CDC)
Description: The CDC strive to protect health and safety, provide reliable health information, and improve health through strong partnerships. The CDC work with partners throughout the United States and the world, and there is a CDC Coordinating Office for Global Health.
Location: Atlanta, GA.
Website: www.cdc.gov

John E. Fogarty International Center (FIC) of the National Institutes of Health (NIH)
Description: As the international component of the U.S. NIH, the FIC addresses global health challenges through innovative and collaborative research and training programs and supports and advances the NIH mission through international partnerships.
Location: Bethesda, MD.
Website: www.fic.nih.gov

Global Fund to Fight AIDS, Tuberculosis, and Malaria
Description: Created to finance a dramatic turnaround in the fight against AIDS, tuberculosis, and malaria, and as a partnership between governments, civil society, the private sector, and affected communities, the Global Fund represents an innovative approach to international

health financing. The Global Fund provides funds around the world, but mostly to sub-Saharan African governments.
Location: Geneva, Switzerland.
Website: www.theglobalfund.org/en/

Institut National de la Santé et de la Recherche Médicale (INSERM)
Description: INSERM is the only French public organization dedicated to biological, medical, and public health research. Its researchers study all human illnesses, whether common or rare. INSERM has a proactive policy of international partnerships.
Location: Paris, France.
Website: www.inserm.fr/en/home.html

Institute of Medicine of the National Academy of Sciences (IOM)
Description: The IOM provides independent, unbiased, evidence-based advice to policy makers, health professionals, industry, and the public. Specific studies advise on how to reduce the burden of disease and disability in developing countries, illuminate emerging threats to international and global health, and emphasize infectious disease.
Location: Washington, DC.
Website: www.iom.edu

International Agency for Research on Cancer (IARC)
Description: The IARC coordinates and conducts research on the causes of human cancer, the mechanisms of carcinogenesis, and the development of scientific strategies for controlling cancer. The IARC is an agency of the World Health Organization.
Location: Lyon, France.
Website: www.iarc.fr

The International Development Research Centre (IDRC)
Description: A Canadian public corporation created to help developing countries use science and technology to find practical, long-term solutions to the social, economic, and environmental problems they are facing, the IDRC provides funds and expert advice to developing-country researchers working to solve critical development problems.
Location: Ottawa, ON. Regional offices in Nairobi, Kenya; Dakar, Senegal; Cairo, Egypt; New Delhi, India; Singapore; and Montevideo, Uruguay.
Website: www.idrc.ca

International Labour Organization (ILO)
Description: The ILO promotes social justice and internationally recognized human and labour rights, and formulates international labour
standards setting minimum standards of basic labour rights: freedom
of association, the right to organize, collective bargaining, abolition of
forced labour, equality of opportunity and treatment, and other standards regulating conditions across the entire spectrum of work-related
issues.
Location: Geneva, Switzerland.
Website: www.ilo.org

International Monetary Fund (IMF)
Description: An organization of 184 countries, the IMF works to foster
global monetary cooperation, secure financial stability, facilitate international trade, promote high employment and sustainable economic
growth, and reduce poverty.
Location: Washington, DC.
Website: www.imf.org

Joint United Nations Programme on HIV/AIDS (UNAIDS)
Description: UNAIDS brings together the efforts and resources of 10
U.N. organizations to the global AIDS response. Co-sponsors of
UNAIDS include UNHCR, UNICEF, WFP, UNDP, UNFPA, UNODC,
ILO, UNESCO, WHO, and the World Bank.
Location: Geneva, Switzerland, with regional support teams in Bang-
kok, Thailand; Johannesburg, South Africa; Dakar, Senegal; Cairo,
Egypt; and Port of Spain, Trinidad and Tobago. UNAIDS operates in
more than 75 countries worldwide.
Website: www.unaids.org/en/

Millennium Challenge Corporation (MCC)
Description: The MCC is the U.S. government body that administers the
Millennium Challenge Account, which provides development assis-
tance to those countries that rule justly, invest in their people, and
encourage economic freedom.
Location: Washington, DC.
Website: www.mca.gov

Office of the U.S. Global AIDS Coordinator (GAC)
Description: The GAC leads in the implementation of the U.S. Presi-

dent's Emergency Plan for AIDS Relief (PEPFAR), which embraces all resources and international activities of the U.S. government to combat the global HIV/AIDS pandemic, including both U.S. bilateral programs and U.S. contributions to multilateral initiatives. PEPFAR puts special emphasis on 15 countries in Africa, Asia, and the Caribbean.
Location: Washington, DC.
Website: www.state.gov/s/gac

Pan American Health Organization (PAHO)
Description: An international public health agency working to improve health and living standards of the countries of the Americas, PAHO is a regional office of the WHO.
Location: Washington, DC.
Website: www.paho.org

Special Programme for Research and Training in Tropical Diseases (TDR)
Description: An independent global program of scientific collaboration, and co-sponsored by UNICEF, UNDP, the World Bank, and the WHO, the TDR aims to help coordinate, support, and influence global efforts to combat a portfolio of major diseases of the poor and disadvantaged through research and training.
Location: Geneva, Switzerland.
Website: www.who.int/tdr

United Kingdom's Department for International Development (DFID)
Description: Part of the U.K. government that manages Britain's aid to poor countries and works to get rid of extreme poverty, the DFID supports long-term programs to help tackle underlying causes of poverty and responds to emergencies, both natural and man-made.
Location: London, England, and East Kilbride (near Glasgow), Scotland, and 25 overseas offices.
Website: www.dfid.gov.uk

United Nations Children's Fund (UNICEF)
Description: UNICEF advocates to protect children's rights, help meet their basic needs, and expand their opportunities to reach their full potential.
Location: New York, NY, with 126 country offices.
Website: www.unicef.org

United Nations Department of Economic and Social Affairs (UNDESA)
Description: UNDESA serves as a vital interface between global policies in the economic, social, and environmental spheres and national action.
Location: New York, NY.
Website: www.un.org/esa/desa

United Nations Development Program (UNDP)
Description: An organization advocating change and connecting countries to knowledge, experience, and resources to help people build a better life, the UNDP works with countries on their own solutions to global and national development challenges.
Location: New York, NY, with 166 country offices.
Website: www.undp.org

United Nations Educational, Scientific, and Cultural Organization (UNESCO)
Description: UNESCO's mission is to contribute to peace and security by promoting collaboration among nations through education, science, and culture in order to further universal respect for justice, for the rule of law, and for the human rights and fundamental freedoms.
Location: Paris, France.
Website: www.unesco.org

United Nations High Commissioner for Refugees (UNHCR)
Description: Mandated to lead and coordinate international action to protect refugees and resolve refugee problems worldwide, the UNHCR has as its primary purpose the safeguarding of the rights and well-being of refugees.
Location: Geneva, Switzerland.
Website: www.unhcr.org/cgi-bin/texis/vtx/home

United Nations Population Fund (UNFPA)
Description: The UNFPA supports countries in using population data for policies and programs to reduce poverty and to ensure that every pregnancy is wanted, every birth is safe, every young person is free of HIV/AIDS, and every girl and woman is treated with dignity and respect.
Location: New York, NY.
Website: www.unfpa.org

United Nations Volunteers
Description: U.N. Volunteers was created to act as a focal point for promoting and harnessing volunteerism for effective development.
Location: Bonn, Germany.
Website: www.unv.org

United Nations World Food Program (WFP)
Description: The WFP is the food aid arm of the U.N. and is oriented towards the objective of eradicating hunger and poverty. The WFP uses food aid to support economic and social development, meet refugee and other emergency food needs, and promote world food security.
Location: Rome, Italy.
Website: www.wfp.org/english/

United States Agency for International Development (USAID)
Description: With the two-pronged purpose of furthering America's foreign policy interests in expanding democracy and free markets while improving the lives of the citizens of the developing world, USAID has been the principal U.S. agency to extend assistance to countries recovering from disaster, trying to escape poverty, and engaging in democratic reforms.
Location: Washington, DC.
Website: www.usaid.gov

United States Peace Corps
Description: The Peace Corps was established to promote world peace and friendship through three goals: (1) helping the people of interested countries to meet their needs for trained men and women, (2) helping promote a better understanding of Americans on the part of the peoples served, and (3) helping promote a better understanding of other peoples on the part of all Americans.
Location: Washington, DC.
Website: www.peacecorps.gov

World Bank
Description: Comprised of the International Bank for Reconstruction and Development (IBRD) and the International Development Association (IDA), the World Bank has 184 member countries. Its mission is global poverty reduction and improvement of living standards. The World Bank provides low-interest loans and interest-free credit and grants to

developing countries for education, health, infrastructure, and communications, as well as many other purposes.
Location: Washington, DC; over 100 offices in member countries
throughout the world.
Website: www.worldbank.org

World Health Organization (WHO)
Description: The WHO's objective is the attainment by all peoples of the
highest possible level of health.
Location: Geneva, Switzerland. Regional offices in Brazzaville, Congo;
Washington, DC; New Delhi, India; Copenhagen, Denmark; Cairo,
Egypt; Manila, Philippines.
Website: www.who.int/en/

Non-Governmental Health Organizations

Sorting through the list of non-governmental organizations (NGOs)
working in global health and medicine that are presented in this chapter
can be overwhelming. Trying to find an appropriate position with one
of them can be even more daunting. First, you should have a sense of the
type of position you are seeking and an awareness of the aspects that
are most important to you. Then, narrow your search for an NGO that
has the health or medical opportunity that best reflects your interests.
You may be able to further narrow your searching by limiting it to
short-, intermediate-, or long-term opportunities, and then to a specific
country or geographical region, religious affiliation, work responsibilities, ability to accommodate family, research opportunities, etc. You
may need to be flexible regarding your criteria, and therefore you must
know what is most important to you. This chapter provides a listing of
over 200 prominent global health NGOs, so hopefully you can find a
suitable fit. Nonetheless, this is not an exhaustive list of organizations
working in global health.

   Generally, it is not difficult to find an NGO in relatively close proxim-
ity to your interests. The country location, the focus of the NGO, and its
philosophy are generally fixed. NGOs are often guided by the people or
organizations that fund their work; the other details, however, can be
variable, and you will need to explore the websites and ask many questions. It is important to examine the mission of the organization by reading about its interests and guiding principles. In addition, speaking
with someone who has had previous success with the organization can

be helpful. You may want to seek work with an NGO in a particular country or an organization with a certain philosophy. If you do not receive a response to your initial inquiry, then be persistent and phone or send an e-mail. Many times, the organization may be able to accommodate you in some way, and the worst outcome is that it declines your services.

There are many NGOs that have a religious affiliation and will often take a volunteer from any religion, provided that the applicant respects the NGO's beliefs and policies. Investigate several different NGOs when you are planning an international opportunity. Often the political situation in a country changes quickly. If the NGO chooses to pull out its personnel, or make other substantial changes, you can be left out in the cold on short notice.

The NGOs listed in this chapter are as diverse as those operating in developing countries. This list is not meant to be all-inclusive, and there are hundreds more – small, large, local, national, and international health organizations – that are not presented. The list in this chapter includes a brief description and contact information for the most prominent organizations working in global health and medicine. Information for NGOs changes often, so be sure to check the websites for the most up-to-date details.

Abt Associates Inc.
Description: A for-profit government and policy research firm, Abt concentrates its work in the areas of international health, economic development, agriculture, natural resources, and socioeconomic issues.
Location: Cambridge, MA.
Website: www.abtassociates.com

Academy for Educational Development (AED)
Description: A not-for-profit organization, the AED addresses human development through education, research, service, and advocacy in many developing countries.
Location: Washington, DC.
Website: www.aed.org

ACDI/VOCA
Description: A not-for-profit organization, ACDI/VOCA promotes broad-based economic growth and the development of civil society in emerging democracies and developing countries.

Location: Washington, DC.
Website: www.acdivoca.org

Action against Hunger (AAH-USA)
Description: A not-for-profit organization, AAH-USA provides relief services, specializing in emergency situations, in more than 40 countries.
Location: New York, NY.
Website: www.actionagainsthunger.org

Action Health
Description: A not-for-profit organization, Action Health works with communities to set up and develop their own health care systems, with local partners in Nigeria, India, Tanzania, and Uganda.
Location: Lagos, Nigeria.
Website: www.actionhealthinc.org

Adventist Development and Relief Agency International (ADRA)
Description: A religiously based organization, ADRA works in food security, economic development, primary health, emergency management, and basic education throughout the world.
Location: Silver Spring, MD.
Website: www.adra.org

AED–Satellite Center for Health Information and Technology
Description: A division of the AED, the Satellite Center provides access to health and medical information services.
Location: Watertown, MA.
Website: www.healthnet.org

African Inland Mission International (AIMI)
Description: A non-denominational Christian missionary-sending agency, the AIMI serves primarily African countries and islands of the Indian Ocean.
Location: Pearl River, NY.
Website: www.aim-us.org

African Medical and Research Foundation (AMREF)
Description: A not-for-profit organization, AMREF seeks to improve the health of people in Africa.

Location: Nairobi, Kenya.
Website: www.amref.org

Africare
Description: A not-for-profit organization, Africare provides assistance to communities across Africa in the areas of food security, health, and HIV/AIDS.
Location: Washington, DC.
Website: www.africare.org

Aga Khan Foundation
Description: A not-for-profit arm of the Aga Khan network, the foundation works to alleviate poverty, hunger, disease, and illiteracy in Africa and Asia.
Location: Washington, DC.
Website: www.akdn.org

AIDS Healthcare Foundation (AHF)
Description: A not-for-profit organization, the AHF brings lifesaving anti-retroviral therapy to developing and resource-poor countries, including South Africa, Uganda, Zambia, India, Swaziland, China, and Ukraine.
Location: Los Angeles, CA.
Website: www.aidshealth.org

Ak'Tenamit
Description: A not-for-profit organization, Ak'Tenamit works to improve access to basic health care and education in Guatemala.
Location: Cuidad de Guatemala, Guatemala.
Website: www.aktenamit.org

Alola Foundation
Description: A not-for-profit organization, Alola works for the advancement of the women of East Timor.
Location: South Melbourne, Australia.
Website: www.alolafoundation.org

Amazon–Africa Aid Organization (3AO)
Description: A not-for-profit organization, 3AO supports Fundacao Esperanca, a Brazilian non-profit organization that provides health care to inhabitants of the Amazon.

Location: Ann Arbor, MI.
Website: www.amazonafrica.org

American College of Surgeons Operation Giving Back
Description: Operation Giving Back provides a comprehensive listing of resources designed to help surgeons find volunteer opportunities best suited to their expertise and interests.
Location: Chicago, IL.
Website: www.operationgivingback.facs.org

American Council for Voluntary International Action (InterAction)
Description: InterAction is an alliance of U.S.-based international development and humanitarian non-governmental organizations.
Location: Washington, DC.
Website: www.interaction.org

American Friends Service Committee
Description: An organization founded by Quakers and co-recipient of the Nobel Peace Prize in 1947, the American Friends Service Committee seeks to understand and address the root causes of poverty, injustice, and war.
Location: Philadelphia, PA, with offices around the world.
Website: www.afsc.org

American Himalayan Foundation (AHF)
Description: A not-for-profit organization, the AHF supports health care projects in the Himalayan region, primarily in Nepal.
Location: San Francisco, CA.
Website: www.himalayan-foundation.org

American International Health Alliance (AIHA)
Description: An international not-for-profit health organization, the AIHA is dedicated to the creation of voluntary health twinning partnerships.
Location: Washington, DC.
Website: www.aiha.com

American Jewish World Service (AJWS)
Description: A religiously affiliated organization, the AJWS seeks to alleviate poverty, hunger, and disease among people in the developing world.

Location: New York, NY.
Website: www.ajws.org

American Leprosy Missions
Description: A not-for-profit organization, American Leprosy Missions
provide medical and comprehensive rehabilitative services to people
affected by leprosy around the world.
Location: Greenville, SC.
Website: www.leprosy.org

American Public Health Association (APHA)
Description: An organization that has sought to influence policies and
set priorities in public health for over 125 years, throughout its history
the APHA has been in the forefront of numerous efforts to prevent disease and promote health.
Location: Washington, DC.
Website: www.apha.org

American Red Cross (Office of International Services)
Description: A not-for-profit organization, the Red Cross helps vulnerable people around the world to prevent, prepare for, and respond to
disasters, complex humanitarian emergencies, and life-threatening
health conditions.
Location: Washington, DC.
Website: www.redcross.org

American Refugee Committee (ARC)
Description: A not-for-profit organization, the ARC works for the sur-
vival, health, and well-being of refugees and displaced persons around
the world.
Location: Minneapolis, MN.
Website: www.archq.org

AMERICARES Foundation
Description: A private, not-for-profit organization, AMERICARES en-
deavours to obtain medicines and medical supplies for people throughout the world. It works in the areas of health, disaster relief, refugees,
and food protection.
Location: Stamford, CT.
Website: www.americares.org

Amigos de las Americas (AMIGOS)
Description: A not-for-profit organization, AMIGOS seeks to train and provide opportunities for high school and college students to participate in service projects in Latin America.
Location: Houston, TX.
Website: www.amigoslink.org

Ann Foundation
Description: A not-for-profit organization, the Ann Foundation seeks to improve the lives of children with disabilities worldwide.
Location: Roslyn, NY.
Website: www.annfoundation.org

Ashoka
Description: An international not-for-profit organization, Ashoka supports public entrepreneurs by connecting them in a professional exchange network.
Location: Arlington, VA.
Website: www.ashoka.org

Bairo Pite Clinic
Description: A not-for-profit clinic, Bairo Pite provides comprehensive community health and medical services in Dili, Timor-Leste.
Location: Dili, Timor-Leste (formerly East Timor, Indonesia).
Website: bairopiteclinic.tripod.com

Bangladesh Rural Advancement Committee (BRAC)
Description: BRAC is involved in the areas of rural banking, education, women's income generation, rural development, and health programs.
Location: Dhaka, Bangladesh.
Website: www.brac.net

Batey Relief Alliance
Description: A not-for-profit organization, Batey Relief helps to create a productive environment through health care and development programs for economically disadvantaged people in the Caribbean.
Location: Brooklyn, NY.
Website: www.bateyrelief.org

Bill and Melinda Gates Foundation
Description: A major not-for-profit organization, the foundation provides grants for global health projects.
Location: Seattle, WA.
Website: www.gatesfoundation.org/globalhealth/

Bridges to Community
Description: A not-for-profit organization, Bridges to Community offers paid and volunteer service-oriented trips to Nicaragua and Kenya.
Location: Ossining, NY.
Website: www.bridgestocommunity.org

Brigada de Salud
Description: A university-affiliated organization, Brigada de Salud provides medical missions in Honduras.
Location: West Lafayette, IN.
Website: www.nursing.purdue.edu/globalinitiatives/honduras.php

Busoga Development Association (BDA)
Description: A not-for-profit Christian organization, the BDA works to empower the poor.
Location: Uganda.
Website: www.busogadev.org

Cameroon Baptist Convention (CBC) Health Board
Description: A religiously affiliated organization, the CBC Health Board supports paying medical volunteers in Cameroon.
Location: Cameroon.
Website: www.cbchealthservices.org

Canadian Council for International Cooperation (CCIC)
Description: A coalition of Canadian voluntary sector organizations, the CCIC is working globally to achieve sustainable human development.
Location: Ottawa, ON.
Website: www.ccic.ca

Canadian Crossroads International (CCI)
Description: A not-for-profit organization, the CCI works to create a more equitable and sustainable world by engaging individuals and organizations.

Location: Toronto, ON.
Website: www.cciorg.ca

Canadian Network for International Surgery (CNIS)
Description: A not-for-profit organization, the CNIS promotes the delivery of essential surgical care to the underprivileged.
Location: Vancouver, BC.
Website: www.cnis.ca

Canadian Physicians for Aid and Relief (CPAR)
Description: A not-for-profit organization, CPAR works in partnership with vulnerable communities and diverse organizations to overcome poverty and build healthy communities in Africa.
Location: Toronto, ON.
Website: www.cpar.ca

Canadian Public Health Association (CPHA)
Description: A not-for-profit organization, the CPHA runs a number of large bilateral public health programs and the Canadian Immunization Initiative.
Location: Ottawa, ON.
Website: www.cpha.ca

Canadian Society for International Health (CSIH)
Description: A not-for-profit organization, the CSIH is for professionals working in the field of global health.
Location: Ottawa, ON.
Website: www.csih.org

Canadian University Services Organization (CUSO)
Description: A not-for-profit organization, CUSO identifies organizations working in the global south that are making real and lasting changes in their own communities.
Location: Ottawa, ON.
Website: www.cuso.org

Cape CARES
Description: A not-for-profit organization, Cape CARES supports paid volunteer medical and dental service trips to Honduras.
Location: Yarmouth, MA.
Website: www.capecares.com

CARE
Description: A large not-for-profit humanitarian organization, CARE fights global poverty, with special focus on working alongside poor women.
Location: Atlanta, GA.
Website: www.care.org

Caritas Internationalis
Description: A not-for-profit confederation of Catholic relief and development organizations, Caritas International was formed to fight poverty.
Location: Vatican City.
Website: www.caritas.org

Carnegie Corporation
Description: A not-for-profit organization, the Carnegie Corporation supports the improvement of maternal health services in Anglophone Africa.
Location: New York, NY.
Website: www.carnegie.org

Carter Center
Description: A not-for-profit organization, the Carter Center is committed to advancing human rights and alleviating unnecessary human suffering.
Location: Atlanta, GA.
Website: www.cartercenter.org

Catholic Medical Mission Board (CMMB)
Description: A not-for-profit organization, the CMMB provides quality health care programs and services to people around the world.
Location: New York, NY.
Website: www.cmmb.org

Catholic Relief Services (CRS)
Description: A large, not-for-profit religiously affiliated organization, CRS promotes human development.
Location: Baltimore, MD.
Website: www.catholicrelief.org

Central American Medical Outreach (CAMO)
Description: A not-for-profit non-denominational Christian organization, CAMO provides medical equipment, community service, supplies, and training to Central America, mostly Honduras.
Location: Orrville, OH.
Website: www.camo.org

Child Family Health International (CFHI)
Description: A not-for-profit organization, CFHI works at the grassroots level to promote the health of the world community.
Location: San Francisco, CA.
Website: www.cfhi.org

Child-to-Child
Description: A not-for-profit international network, Child-to-Child promotes children's participation in health and development.
Location: London, England.
Website: www.child-to-child.org/form.html

Children International
Description: A not-for-profit organization, Children International provides medical care, counselling, and materials to children in 13 countries.
Location: Kansas City, MS.
Website: www.children.org

Children's AIDS Fund
Description: A not-for-profit organization, the Children's AIDS Fund provides care, services, resources, referrals, and education to HIV-affected children and their families.
Location: Sterling, VA.
Website: www.childrensaidsfund.org

Children's Cross Connection International (CCCI)
Description: A not-for-profit Judeo-Christian organization, CCCI provides medical services and teaching in Ethiopia and El Salvador.
Location: Fayetteville, GA.
Website: www.cccinternational.org

Christian Children's Fund of Canada (CCFC)
Description: A not-for-profit organization, the CCFC is committed to helping children and their families around the globe living in poverty.
Location: Toronto, ON.
Website: www.ccfcanada.ca

Christian Emergency Relief Teams International (CERT)
Description: A not-for-profit organization, the CERT seeks to alleviate human suffering by providing medical and dental services in remote locations.
Location: Crossville, TN.
Website: www.certinternational.org

Christian Medical and Dental Society/Associations (CMDA)
Description: A not-for-profit organization, CMDA provides international short-term mission opportunities for medical, dental, and other health care professionals.
Location: Bristol, TN.
Website: www.cmda.org

Community Information and Epidemiological Technologies International (CIET)
Description: An international group of epidemiologists and social scientists, CIET brings scientific research methods to local government and community levels.
Location: New York, NY.
Website: www.ciet.org

CONCERN Worldwide (U.S.)
Description: A not-for-profit organization, CONCERN Worldwide implements development programs that focus on health, nutrition, and HIV/AIDS in many poor countries.
Location: New York, NY.
Website: www.concernusa.org

Constella Group
Description: A for-profit organization, the Constella Group specializes in the design and implementation of public health and social programs for developing countries.
Location: Durham, NC.
Website: www.constellagroup.com/international-development/

Council on Health Research for Development (COHRED)
Description: A not-for-profit organization, COHRED provides a voice for
Health Research for Development to strengthen southern institutions.
Location: Geneva, Switzerland.
Website: www.cohred.org

Cross Cultural Solutions (CCS)
Description: A not-for-profit organization, CCS offers volunteer abroad
programs in health clinics and hospitals in 10 countries.
Location: New Rochelle, NY.
Website: www.crossculturalsolutions.org

Curamericas
Description: A not-for-profit organization, Curamericas conducts health
work in Bolivia, Guatemala, Haiti, and Mexico.
Location: Raleigh, NC.
Website: www.curamericas.org

CURE International
Description: A not-for-profit organization, CURE establishes rehabilita-
tion hospitals for disabled children in developing countries.
Location: Lemoyne, PA.
Website: www.cureinternational.org

David and Lucile Packard Foundation
Description: A not-for-profit organization, the foundation provides
grants to organizations in several program areas.
Location: Los Altos, CA.
Website: www.packard.org

Dignitas International
Description: A not-for-profit humanitarian organization, Dignitas pro-
vides immediate and sustainable long-term solutions for individuals
and communities living with HIV/AIDS.
Location: Toronto, ON.
Website: www.dignitasinternational.org

DOCARE International, NFP
Description: A not-for-profit organization, DOCARE provides osteopathic medical outreach to people in remote areas of western hemisphere countries.

Location: East Dundee, IL.
Website: www.docareintl.org

Doctors for Global Health (DGH)
Description: A not-for-profit organization, DGH promotes health and
human rights throughout the world.
Location: Decatur, GA.
Website: www.dghonline.org

Doctors of the World (DOW)
Description: A not-for-profit organization, DOW provides training, ca-
pacity building, clinical services, and advocacy to address health and
human rights issues.
Location: New York, NY.
Website: www.doctorsoftheworld.org

Doctors without Borders (Médecins sans Frontières)
Description: A not-for-profit medical humanitarian organization,
Doctors without Borders delivers emergency aid to people in more
than 70 countries.
Location: Main headquarters in Paris, France; U.S. headquarters in New
York, NY.
Website: www.doctorswithoutborders.org

Earthwatch Institute
Description: A not-for-profit organization, Earthwatch offers opportuni-
ties in global health work.
Location: San Francisco, CA.
Website: www.earthwatch.org

Edna McConnell Clark Foundation
Description: A not-for-profit organization, the foundation supports
interventions and research efforts to control onchocerciasis, schistoso-
miasis, and blinding trachoma.
Location: New York, NY.
Website: www.emcf.org

Elizabeth Glaser Pediatric AIDS Foundation
Description: A not-for-profit organization, the foundation conducts
research programs and advocacy efforts to fight against pediatric HIV/
AIDS in the developing world.

Location: Washington, DC.
Website: www.pedaids.org

EngenderHealth
Description: A not-for-profit organization, EngenderHealth works to achieve sustainable health delivery systems and to enable people to have healthier lives.
Location: New York, NY.
Website: www.engenderhealth.org

Episcopal Medical Missions Foundation (EMMF)
Description: A not-for-profit religiously affiliated organization, the EMMF conducts short-term projects in the Philippines, Africa, Dominican Republic, Ecuador, Jamaica, Honduras, and Mexico.
Location: Austin, TX.
Website: www.emmf.com

Episcopal Relief and Development (ERD)
Description: A not-for-profit religiously affiliated organization, ERD provides emergency assistance after disasters, rebuilds communities, and helps children and families climb out of poverty.
Location: New York, NY.
Website: www.er-d.org

Esperanca
Description: A not-for-profit organization, Esperanca provides health services to people in Bolivia, Mozambique, and Nicaragua.
Location: Phoenix, AZ.
Website: www.esperanca.org

Family Care International
Description: A not-for-profit organization, Family Care is committed to improving maternal health.
Location: New York, NY.
Website: www.familycareintl.org

Family Health International (FHI)
Description: A large, not-for-profit organization, FHI manages research and field activities to meet the public health needs of the world's most vulnerable people.
Location: Research Triangle Park, NC.
Website: www.fhi.org

Feed the Children
Description: A not-for-profit organization, Feed the Children supplies food, medicine, medical equipment, and other necessities to people in more than 20 countries.
Location: Oklahoma City, OK.
Website: www.feedthechildren.org

Fellowship of Associates of Medical Evangelism (FAME)
Description: A not-for-profit religiously affiliated organization, FAME conducts short-term medical missions.
Location: Indianapolis, IN.
Website: www.fameworld.org

Filipino-American Medical (FAM)
Description: A not-for-profit organization, FAM brings American health care providers to serve the poor in the Philippines.
Location: New York, NY.
Website: ifami.com

Flying Doctors of America (FDA)
Description: A not-for-profit organization of health care providers and non-medical support volunteers, FDA conducts short-term medical trips around the world.
Location: Cartersville, GA.
Website: www.fdoamerica.org

Flying Samaritans International (FSI)
Description: A not-for-profit organization, FSI operates medical clinics in Baja, California, and Mexico.
Location: Lake Forest, CA.
Website: www.flyingsamaritans.org

Ford Foundation
Description: A large not-for-profit organization, the Ford Foundation provides grants to strengthen democratic values, reduce poverty and injustice, promote international cooperation, and advance human achievement.
Location: New York, NY.
Website: www.fordfound.org

Foundation Center
Description: A not-for-profit organization, the Center strengthens the
non-profit sector by advancing knowledge about U.S. philanthropy.
Location: New York, NY.
Website: foundationcenter.org

Foundation Human Nature USA (FHNUSA)
Description: A not-for-profit organization, FHNUSA conducts commu-
nity-based rural health and development projects in Ecuador and
Ghana.
Location: Los Angeles, CA.
Website: www.fhnusa.org

Friends of the Orphans (Nuestros Pequeños Hermanos)
Description: A not-for-profit religiously affiliated organization, Friends
of the Orphans provides shelter, health care, and education to or-
phaned children in Latin America and the Caribbean.
Location: Arlington Heights, IL.
Website: www.friendsoftheorphans.org

Friends United Meeting (FUM)
Description: A not-for-profit religiously affiliated organization, FUM
works in areas of public health, population planning, and nutrition.
Location: Richmond, IN.
Website: www.fum.org

Friends without a Border
Description: A not-for-profit organization, Friends without a Border
supports Angkor Hospital for Children in Siem Reap, Cambodia.
Location: New York, NY.
Website: www.fwab.org

A Glimmer of Hope Foundation
Description: A not-for-profit organization, the foundation focuses on
making a sustainable difference in the lives of rural poor of Ethiopia.
Location: Austin, TX.
Website: www.aglimmerofhope.org

Global Healing
Description: A not-for-profit organization, Global Healing establishes

modern health care programs in developing countries throughout the world.
Location: Orinda, CA.
Website: www.globalhealing.org

Global Health Action
Description: A not-for-profit organization, Global Health Action creates sustainable health programs and trains health professionals in several developing countries.
Location: Decatur, GA.
Website: www.globalhealthaction.org

Global Health Education Consortium (GHEC)
Description: A not-for-profit organization, the GHEC focuses on global health education and conducts an annual conference.
Location: San Francisco, CA.
Website: www.globalhealth-ec.org

Global Health Ministries
Description: A not-for-profit religiously affiliated organization, Global Health Ministries supports the health care work of Lutheran churches in developing countries.
Location: Minneapolis, Minnesota.
Website: www.ghm.org

Global Health through Education, Training, and Service (GHETS)
Description: A not-for-profit organization, GHETS is dedicated to improving health in developing countries through innovations in education and service.
Location: Attleboro, MA.
Website: www.ghets.org

Global Lawyers and Physicians (GLP)
Description: A not-for-profit organization, GLP focuses on health and human rights issues.
Location: Boston, MA.
Website: www.glphr.org

Global Outreach
Description: A not-for-profit religiously affiliated organization, Global

Outreach works in agriculture and crop production in developing countries, and spreads Christian values.
Location: Tupelo, MS.
Website: www.globaloutreach.org

Global Service Corps
Description: A not-for-profit organization, the Global Service Corps organizes short-term opportunities for working in Thailand and Tanzania.
Location: San Francisco, CA.
Website: www.globalservicecorps.org

Global Volunteers
Description: A not-for-profit organization, Global Volunteers provides short-term health and education opportunities in several countries.
Location: St Paul, MN.
Website: www.globalvolunteers.org

Grokha Association of Social Health (GASH)
Description: A not-for-profit organization, GASH provides health services in rural Nepal.
Location: Katmandu, Nepal.
Website: www.geocities.com/gash_nepal

GuluWalk
Description: A not-for-profit organization, GuluWalk brings funding and awareness to the plight of orphans in Northern Uganda.
Location: Toronto, ON.
Website: www.guluwalk.com

Hands Together
Description: A not-for-profit religiously affiliated organization, Hands Together improves the quality of life for poor people in Haiti through education and health.
Location: Springfield, MA.
Website: www.handstogether.org

Healing Hands International
Description: A not-for-profit organization, Healing Hands addresses worldwide disasters and needs in developing countries by distributing medical supplies and resources.

Location: Nashville, TN.
Website: www.hhi-aid.org

Healing the Children Northeast (HTCNE)
Description: A not-for-profit organization, HTCNE provides short-term medical treatment programs around the world.
Location: New Milford, CT.
Website: www.htcne.org

HealthCare Volunteer
Description: A not-for-profit organization, HealthCare Volunteer connects medical volunteers with thousands of volunteering opportunities all over the world.
Location: Los Angeles, CA.
Website: www.healthcarevolunteer.com

Healthlink Worldwide
Description: A not-for-profit organization, Healthlink mobilizes innovative knowledge and communication processes and empowers people to voice their health needs and have those voices heard.
Location: London, England.
Website: www.healthlink.org.uk

HealthPartners
Description: A not-for-profit organization, HealthPartners develops local health care delivery programs in Uganda.
Location: Minneapolis, MN.
Website: www.healthpartners.com

HealthWrights
Description: A not-for-profit organization, HealthWrights works to advance health, basic rights, and social equality among disadvantaged persons.
Location: Palo Alto, CA.
Website: www.healthwrights.org

Health Alliance International (HAI)
Description: A not-for-profit organization, HAI supports the development of equity-oriented policies and public-sector health systems for a world with universal access to quality health care.

Location: Seattle, WA.
Website: depts.washington.edu/haiuw/

Health for Humanity
Description: A not-for-profit organization, Health for Humanity conducts blindness prevention, maternal and child health, and international physician exchange projects in several developing countries.
Location: Wilmette, IL.
Website: www.healthforhumanity.org

Health Frontiers
Description: A not-for-profit organization, Health Frontiers seeks international health and child development opportunities.
Location: Kenyon, MN.
Website: www.healthfrontiers.org

Health Unlimited
Description: A not-for-profit organization, Health Unlimited supports communities living amidst conflict.
Location: London, United Kingdom.
Website: www.healthunlimited.org

Health Volunteers Overseas
Description: A not-for-profit organization, Health Volunteers Overseas seeks to improve the availability and quality of health care in developing countries through training and education.
Location: Washington, DC.
Website: www.hvousa.org

Helen Keller International (HKI)
Description: A not-for-profit organization, HKI works in establishing nutrition and eye health programs in partnership with host countries.
Location: New York, NY.
Website: www.hki.org

HELPS International
Description: A not-for-profit organization, HELPS works to improve health care, education, and development in Guatemala.
Location: Addison, TX.
Website: www.helpsintl.org

Hesperian Foundation
Description: A not-for-profit organization, the Hesperian Foundation publishes books for community health workers in rural settings.
Location: Berkeley, CA.
Website: www.hesperian.org

Himalayan HealthCare
Description: A not-for-profit organization, Himalayan HealthCare provides primary health care, community education, and income-generating projects in rural Nepal.
Location: New York, NY.
Website: www.himalayan-healthcare.org

HOPE Worldwide
Description: A not-for-profit organization, HOPE Worldwide provides health and education programs to poor people in many developing countries.
Location: Wayne, PA.
Website: www.hopeww.org

Hôpital Bon Samaritain (HBS) Foundation
Description: A not-for-profit organization, the HBS Foundation supports the Hôpital Bon Samaritain, a primary health care centre, in rural Haiti.
Location: Lake Worth, FL.
Website: www.hbslimbe.org

Human Rights Watch
Description: A large, not-for-profit organization, Human Rights Watch conducts human rights activities around the world.
Location: Chicago, IL.
Website: www.hrw.org

Idealist.org
Description: A not-for-profit organization, Idealist.org promotes the sharing of ideas, information, and resources to help build a world where all people can live free, dignified, and productive lives.
Location: New York, NY.
Website: www.idealist.org

Inter Pares
Description: A not-for-profit organization, Inter Pares works in social and economic justice issues.
Location: Ottawa, ON.
Website: www.interpares.ca

Interaction
Description: A not-for-profit organization, Interaction maintains an alliance of U.S.-based international development and humanitarian non-governmental organizations.
Location: Washington, DC.
Website: www.interaction.org

International AIDS Vaccine Initiative (IAVI)
Description: A global not-for-profit organization, the IAVI is working to speed the search for a vaccination to prevent HIV infection and AIDS.
Location: New York, NY.
Website: www.iavi.org

International Center for AIDS Care and Treatment Programs (ICAP)
Description: A not-for-profit organization, the ICAP focuses on service delivery, research, and training and education in resource-limited settings to help address the HIV/AIDS epidemic.
Location: New York, NY.
Website: www.columbia-icap.org

International Center for Research on Women (ICRW)
Description: A not-for-profit organization, the ICRW works on issues affecting women's economic, health, and social status in India and Uganda.
Location: Washington, DC.
Website: www.icrw.org

International Clinical Epidemiology Network (INCLEN)
Description: A not-for-profit organization, INCLEN promotes health care delivery by training physicians in developing countries and linking health research to policy making.
Location: Philadelphia, PA.
Website: www.inclen.org

International Council on Social Welfare (ICSW)
Description: A not-for-profit organization, the ICSW seeks to promote social development.
Location: Montreal, QC.
Website: www.iswc.org

International Epidemiology Institute (IEI)
Description: The IEI provides state-of-the-science expertise in addressing complex biomedical issues.
Location: Rockville, MD.
Website: www.iei.ws

International Federation of Red Cross and Red Crescent Societies (IFRC)
Description: A not-for-profit global humanitarian organization, the IFRC provides assistance without discrimination as to nationality, race, religious beliefs, class, or political opinions.
Location: Geneva, Switzerland.
Website: www.ifrc.org

International Health Organization (IHO)
Description: A not-for-profit organization, the IHO is dedicated to improving the health and well-being of underserved people in rural South Asia.
Location: Boston, MA.
Website: www.ihousa.org

International HIV/AIDS Alliance
Description: A not-for-profit organization, the Alliance is working towards supporting effective community responses to HIV/AIDS in several developing countries.
Location: Brighton, United Kingdom.
Website: www.aidsalliance.org

International Medical Corps (IMC)
Description: A not-for-profit organization, the IMC conducts training programs and delivers essential health services.
Location: Santa Monica, CA.
Website: www.imcworldwide.org

International Medical Equipment Collaborative of America (IMEC)
Description: A not-for-profit organization, the IMEC provides quality tools to doctors and nurses in several developing countries.
Location: North Andover, MA.
Website: www.imecamerica.org

International Medical Services for Health (INMED)
Description: A not-for-profit organization, INMED increases resources for community development by bringing together health care and education for child-centred strategies.
Location: Sterling, VA.
Website: www.inmed.org

International Medical Volunteers Association (IMVA)
Description: A not-for-profit organization, the IMVA seeks to connect international medical volunteers.
Location: Woodville, MA.
Website: www.imva.org

International Physicians for the Prevention of Nuclear War (IPPNW)
Description: A not-for-profit organization, IPPNW seeks to prevent nuclear war and abolish nuclear weapons, and to reduce armed conflict around the world.
Location: Cambridge, MA.
Website: www.ippnw.org

International Planned Parenthood Federation (IPPF)
Description: A not-for-profit corporation, the IPPF represents a federation of autonomous national family planning associations.
Location: New York, NY.
Website: www.ippfwhr.org

International Relief Teams (IRT)
Description: A not-for-profit organization, IRT provides medical relief during natural disasters and other crises and distributes medical supplies.
Location: San Diego, CA.
Website: www.irteams.org

International Rescue Committee (IRC)
Description: A large not-for-profit organization, the IRC provides relief and services for refugees and displaced persons in several developing countries.
Location: New York, NY.
Website: www.theirc.org

International Service Learning (ISL)
Description: A not-for-profit organization, the ISL organizes field experiences in health care services in several developing countries.
Location: Corpus Christi, TX.
Website: www.islonline.org

International Women's Health Coalition (IWHC)
Description: A not-for-profit organization, the IWHC is dedicated to improving women's reproductive health in developing countries.
Location: New York, NY.
Website: www.iwhc.org

International Youth Foundation (IYF)
Description: A not-for-profit organization, the IYF seeks to improve the conditions and prospects for young people where they live, learn, work, and play.
Location: Baltimore, MD.
Website: www.ifynet.org

Interplast
Description: A not-for-profit organization, Interplast provides reconstructive surgery for children with congenital deformities in developing countries.
Location: Mountain View, CA.
Website: www.interplast.org

IntraHealth International
Description: A not-for-profit organization, IntraHealth International seeks to improve the health and well-being of women and their families around the world by improving the quality and accessibility of health care services.
Location: Chapel Hill, NC.
Website: www.intrahealth.org

Ipas
Description: A not-for-profit organization, Ipas seeks to increase women's ability to exercise their sexual and reproductive rights and to reduce abortion-related deaths and injuries.
Location: Chapel Hill, NC.
Website: www.ipas.org

JHPIEGO (Affiliate of Johns Hopkins University)
Description: A not-for-profit organization, JHPIEGO seeks to enhance the quality of health care services for women and families, with a focus on training and support for health care providers.
Location: Baltimore, MD.
Website: www.jhpiego.org

John D. and Catherine T. MacArthur Foundation
Description: A not-for-profit organization, the foundation provides grants for sustainable development and for population and reproductive health.
Location: Chicago, IL.
Website: www.macfound.org

John Snow, Inc. (JSI)
Description: A for-profit organization, JSI seeks to improve the health of individuals and communities in developing countries.
Location: Boston, MA.
Website: www.jsi.com

Kaiser Family Foundation
Description: A not-for-profit organization, the foundation focuses on the major health care issues facing the United States, with a growing role in global health.
Location: Menlo Park, CA.
Website: www.kff.org

W.K. Kellogg Foundation
Description: A not-for-profit organization, the foundation provides grants for health work in developing countries.
Location: Battle Creek, MI.
Website: www.wkkf.org

Lalmba
Description: A not-for-profit organization, Lalmba provides health care services in East Africa.
Location: Arvada, CO.
Website: www.lalmba.org

Liga International (Flying Doctors of Mercy)
Description: A not-for-profit organization, Liga provides surgical treatment to people around the world.
Location: Rialto, CA.
Website: www.ligainternational.org

Luke Society
Description: A not-for-profit religiously affiliated organization of Christian health and business professionals, the Luke Society is dedicated to medical missions.
Location: Sioux Falls, SD.
Website: www.lukesociety.org

Lutheran World Relief (LWR)
Description: A not-for-profit religiously affiliated organization, LWR seeks lasting solutions to poverty and injustice.
Location: Baltimore, MD.
Website: www.lwr.org

Malaika Project
Description: A not-for-profit international collaboration, the Malaika Project seeks to improve the living conditions of people in western Tanzania.
Location: Chicopee, MA.
Website: www.malaikaproject.org

Management Sciences for Health (MSH)
Description: A not-for-profit organization, MSH supports large-scale responses to priority health problems in developing countries.
Location: Cambridge, MA.
Website: www.msh.org

MAP International
Description: A not-for-profit religiously affiliated organization, MAP

donates medicines and medical supplies through Christian hospitals and clinics.
Location: Brunswick, GA.
Website: www.map.org

Maryknoll Lay Missioners (MLM)
Description: A not-for-profit Catholic organization, MLM conducts mission work with refugees, orphans, and sick people around the world.
Location: Maryknoll, NY.
Website: www.mklaymissioners.org

Medical Ambassadors International (MAI)
Description: A not-for-profit religiously affiliated organization, MAI is working to improve the health and living standards of people in poor areas of the world.
Location: Modesto, CA.
Website: www.med-amb.org

Medical Benevolence Foundation (MBF)
Description: A not-for-profit organization, the MBF provides development assistance, training, and program support in basic medical and dental care to selected overseas hospitals.
Location: Houston, TX.
Website: www.mbfoundation.org

Medical Care Development (MCD)
Description: A not-for-profit organization, MCD provides technical assistance to support and improve the health and socioeconomic status of people in developing countries.
Location: Augusta, ME.
Website: www.mcd.org

Medical Education Cooperation with Cuba (MEDICC)
Description: A not-for-profit organization, MEDICC offers medical education and training in Cuba.
Location: Atlanta, GA.
Website: www.medicc.org

Medical, Eye and Dental International Care Organization (MEDICO)
Description: A not-for-profit organization, MEDICO provides free

health and educational services to impoverished people in Latin America, and conducts short-term medical missions.
Location: Georgetown, TX.
Website: www.medico.org

Medical Ministry International (MMInt)
Description: A not-for-profit religiously affiliated organization, MMInt provides opportunities for short-term medical projects.
Location: Allen, TX.
Website: www.mmint.org

Medical Mission International (MMI)
Description: A not-for-profit organization, MMI provides surgical procedures and skills to the needy in rural El Salvador.
Location: Palm Harbor, FL.
Website: www.medicalmissioninternational.org

Medical Missions for Children (MMC)
Description: A not-for-profit organization, MMC seeks to improve health care for medically underserved communities through telemedicine.
Location: Paterson, NJ.
Website: www.mmissions.org

Medical Services Corporation International (MSCI)
Description: MSCI is a not-for-profit health management firm engaged in a variety of health care activities.
Location: Arlington, VA.
Website: www.mscionline.com

Medicine for Peace
Description: A not-for-profit organization, Medicine for Peace provides health care services for mothers and children who are victims of war in Iraq, Bosnia, Haiti, and El Salvador.
Location: Washington, DC.
Website: www.medicineforpeace.org

MedShare International
Description: A not-for-profit organization, MedShare collects unused surplus medical supplies and equipment and distributes them to hospitals and medical teams worldwide.

Location: Decatur, GA.
Website: www.medshare.org

Mercy Corps
Description: A not-for-profit organization, Mercy Corps provides emergency relief that assists people afflicted by conflict or disaster and community development in countries worldwide.
Location: Portland, OR.
Website: www.mercycorps.org

Mercy Ships
Description: A not-for-profit organization, Mercy Ships operates hospital ships as a platform for providing specialized surgeries to patients in the developing world.
Location: Lindale, TX.
Website: www.mercyships.org

Merlin
Description: A not-for-profit organization, Merlin provides health care and medical relief for vulnerable people in natural disasters, conflict, and health system collapse.
Location: London, England.
Website: www.merlin.org.uk

Mexican Medical Ministries (MMM)
Description: A not-for-profit interdenominational religious organization, MMM provides health care to the people of Mexico.
Location: Chula Vista, CA.
Website: www.mexicanmedical.com

Minnesota International Health Volunteers (MIHV)
Description: A not-for-profit organization, MIHV addresses the health needs of people in Uganda.
Location: Minneapolis, MN.
Website: www.mihv.org

Mission Aviation Fellowship (MAF)
Description: A not-for-profit religiously affiliated organization, MAF provides flights into remote regions of the world, together with communication services and learning technologies.

Location: Nampa, ID.
Website: www.maf.org

Mission Doctors Association (MDA)
Description: A not-for-profit religiously affiliated organization, MDA recruits, trains, sends, and supports Catholic doctors to serve at mission hospitals and clinics around the world.
Location: Los Angeles, CA.
Website: www.missiondoctors.org

Mountain Mover's Missions International
Description: A not-for-profit organization, Mountain Mover's provides medical assistance, human rights support, and civil aid to the people of Honduras.
Location: Danli, Honduras.
Website: www.geocities.com/clinica_eya

Near East Foundation (NEF)
Description: A not-for-profit organization, the NEF promotes sustainable development, mainly in the Middle East and Northern Africa.
Location: New York, NY.
Website: www.nefdev.org

NET CORPS
Description: An initiative of six not-for-profit Canadian organizations, NET CORPS helps develop training for youth in developing countries to acquire, build, and spread telecommunications infrastructure.
Location: Montréal, QC.
Website: www.netcorps-cyberjeunes.org

North-South Institute (NSI)
Description: A not-for-profit research institute, NSI is dedicated to eradicating global poverty and enhancing social justice through research that promotes international cooperation, democratic governance, and conflict prevention.
Location: Ottawa, ON.
Website: www.nsi-ins.ca/english/default.asp

Northwest Medical Teams International (NWMT)
Description: A not-for-profit organization, NWMT recruits and sends

volunteer teams to disaster areas in developing countries to provide medical care, supplies, and health education.
Location: Portland, OR.
Website: www.nwmedicalteams.org

Omni Med
Description: A not-for-profit organization, Omni Med organizes short-term medical work in Belize, Guyana, and Kenya.
Location: Weban, MA.
Website: www.omnimed.org

Open Society Foundation (Soros Foundation)
Description: A not-for-profit organization, the foundation provides grants to promote public health and women's rights.
Location: New York, NY.
Website: www.soros.org

Operation Blessing International Relief and Development
Description: A not-for-profit organization, Operation Blessing implements programs that focus on disaster relief, medical aid, hunger relief, and community development in developing countries.
Location: Virginia Beach, VA.
Website: www.ob.org

Operation Crossroads Africa
Description: A not-for-profit organization, Operation Crossroads offers a cross-cultural exchange program.
Location: New York, NY.
Website: operationcrossroadsafrica.org

Operation Rainbow
Description: A not-for-profit organization, Operation Rainbow provides free plastic and orthopedic surgery to children in medically underserved countries around the world.
Location: Oakland, CA.
Website: www.operationrainbow.org

Operation Serve International (OSI)
Description: A not-for-profit religiously affiliated organization, OSI organizes short health-related projects in Egypt and Mexico.

Location: Fairfield, OH.
Website: www.operationserve.org

Operation Smile
Description: A not-for-profit organization, Operation Smile provides free facial surgery to children with congenital deformities throughout the world.
Location: Norfolk, VA.
Website: www.operationsmile.org

OXFAM
Description: A large not-for-profit organization, OXFAM seeks to create lasting solutions to global poverty, hunger, and social injustice.
Location: Oxford, England, and Boston, MA.
Website: www.oxfamamerica.org

Palestine Children's Relief Fund (PCRF)
Description: A not-for-profit organization, the PCRF arranges free medical care in the United States for injured and sick youth in the Middle East who cannot be treated locally.
Location: Kent, OH.
Website: www.pcrf.net

Partners for Development (PFD)
Description: A not-for-profit organization, PFD works to improve living standards in Bosnia-Herzegovina, Cambodia, and Nigeria.
Location: Silver Spring, MD.
Website: www.pfd.org

Partners in Health (PIH)
Description: A not-for-profit organization, PIH provides medical care and services to poor people in Haiti, Peru, and Rwanda.
Location: Boston, MA.
Website: www.pih.org

Partners of the Americas
Description: A not-for-profit organization, Partners undertakes health and development work throughout Latin America.
Location: Washington, DC.
Website: www.partners.net

Pathfinder International
Description: A not-for-profit organization, Pathfinder provides access to quality family planning and reproductive health information and services throughout the world.
Location: Watertown, MA.
Website: www.pathfind.org

Peacework
Description: A not-for-profit organization, Peacework offers short-term volunteer opportunities to promote solutions to poverty and disparity through development, education, health, and service.
Location: Blacksburg, VA.
Website: www.peacework.org

Pew Charitable Trusts (PCT)
Description: A not-for-profit organization, the PCT supports the public interest by providing information, advancing policy solutions, and supporting civic life.
Location: Philadelphia, PA.
Website: www.pewtrusts.com

Physicians for Human Rights (PHR)
Description: A not-for-profit organization, PHR promotes health by protecting human rights.
Location: Cambridge, MA.
Website: www.phrusa.org

Physicians for Peace Foundation (PPF)
Description: A not-for-profit organization, the PPF provides medical education in a variety of specialties to health care professionals and conducts medical missions to developing countries.
Location: Norfolk, VA.
Website: www.physiciansforpeace.org

Physicians for Social Responsibility (PSR)
Description: A not-for-profit organization, PSR seeks to stop nuclear war and slow, stop, and reverse toxic degradation of the environment and global warming.
Location: Washington, DC.
Website: www.psr.org

PLAN International
Description: A not-for-profit organization, PLAN helps families reduce poverty and better their health through interventions in HIV/AIDS and child survival.
Location: Warwick, RI.
Website: www.planusa.org

Planned Parenthood Federation of America
Description: A not-for-profit organization, Planned Parenthood provides sexuality education, family planning, and reproductive services to women, adolescents, and migrants.
Location: New York, NY.
Website: www.ppfa.org

Plasticos Foundation
Description: A not-for-profit organization, Plasticos provides services to correct birth defects, congenital malformation, and traumatic disfigurement in developing countries.
Location: Huntington Beach, CA.
Website: www.plasticosfoundation.org

Population Council
Description: A not-for-profit organization, the Population Council improves the reproductive health of people in developing countries.
Location: New York, NY.
Website: www.popcouncil.org

Population Services International (PSI)
Description: A not-for-profit organization, PSI uses social marketing to deliver health information, services, and products to enable people to lead healthier lives.
Location: Washington, DC.
Website: www.psi.org

PRISMA
Description: A not-for-profit organization, PRISMA works with poor and vulnerable populations to implement programs for economic welfare and social development.
Location: Lima, Peru.
Website: www.prisma.org.pe

Program for Appropriate Technology in Health (PATH)
Description: A not-for-profit organization, PATH seeks to create sustainable solutions to improve health in developing countries.
Location: Seattle, WA.
Website: www.path.org

Progressio
Description: A not-for-profit organization, Progressio works for justice and the eradication of poverty in developing countries.
Location: London, England.
Website: www.ciir.org

Project Concern International
Description: A not-for-profit organization, Project Concern seeks to provide access to health resources and promotes development through community-based solutions.
Location: San Diego, CA.
Website: www.projectconcern.org

Project HOPE (People-to-People Health Foundation)
Description: A not-for-profit organization, Project HOPE conducts medical training, health education, and humanitarian assistance in developing countries.
Location: Millwood, VA.
Website: www.projecthope.org

Project ORBIS International
Description: A not-for-profit organization, Project ORBIS provides surgical missions and trains health care providers in developing countries.
Location: New York, NY.
Website: www.orbis.org

Project Peds
Description: A not-for-profit organization, Project Peds is dedicated to building a new hospital for the local population in Matara, Sri Lanka.
Location: West Hollywood, CA.
Website: www.slprojectpeds.org/cs

Recovered Medical Equipment for the Developing World (REMEDY)
Description: A not-for-profit organization, REMEDY seeks to collect and recycle medical supplies for donations to developing countries.

Location: New Haven, CT.
Website: www.remedyinc.org

Relief International
Description: A not-for-profit humanitarian organization, Relief International provides emergency relief, rehabilitation, development assistance, and program services.
Location: Los Angeles, CA.
Website: www.ri.org

Remote Area Medical Volunteer Corps (RAMVC)
Description: A not-for-profit organization, RAMVC conducts short-term medical missions to remote areas of the world.
Location: Knoxville, TN.
Website: www.ramusa.org

Robert Wood Johnson Foundation
Description: A large not-for-profit organization, the foundation is devoted to improving health and health care.
Location: Princeton, NJ.
Website: www.rwjf.org

Rockefeller Foundation
Description: A not-for-profit organization, the foundation provides grants to promote health equity and food security.
Location: New York, NY.
Website: www.rockfound.org

Rotary Foundation of Rotary International
Description: A large not-for-profit organization, the foundation supplies humanitarian services and health and education to developing countries.
Location: Evanston, IL.
Website: www.rotary.org

Save the Children Federation
Description: A not-for-profit organization, Save the Children seeks to mobilize assistance to help children recover from the effects of war, conflict, and natural disasters.
Location: Westport, CT.
Website: www.savethechildren.org

SIM USA
Description: A not-for-profit non-denominational religious organization, SIM USA provides humanitarian services to people around the world.
Location: Charlotte, NC.
Website: www.sim.org

Simeus Foundation
Description: A not-for-profit organization, the foundation seeks to improve the standard of living for the poor in Haiti by providing medical care, clean water, education, nutritional services, and clothing.
Location: Mansfield, TX.
Website: www.simeusfoundation.org

Stephen Lewis Foundation
Description: A not-for-profit organization, the foundation provides care to women who are ill and struggling to survive; assists orphans and other AIDS-affected children; supports heroic grandmothers who almost single-handedly care for their orphan grandchildren; and supports associations of people living with HIV/AIDS.
Location: Toronto, ON.
Website: www.stephenlewisfoundation.org

Support for International Change (SIChange)
Description: A not-for-profit organization, SIChange provides HIV testing, conducts HIV/AIDS awareness campaigns, and provides health worker training in Tanzania.
Location: Arusha, Tanzania.
Website: www.sichange.org/home/

Surgical Eye Expeditions International (SEEI)
Description: A not-for-profit organization, SEEI provides medical, surgical, and educational services by volunteer ophthalmic surgeons to blind individuals worldwide.
Location: Santa Barbara, CA.
Website: www.seeintl.org

Surgicorps International
Description: A not-for-profit organization, Surgicorps is dedicated to providing reconstructive surgery for children in less-developed countries.

Location: Glenshaw, PA.
Website: www.surgicorps.org

United Nations Foundation
Description: A not-for-profit organization, the foundation seeks to enable people to support United Nations causes and activities.
Location: Washington, DC.
Website: www.unfoundation.org

United Planet
Description: A not-for-profit organization, United Planet seeks to foster cross-cultural understanding and fellowship and enhance social and economic prosperity among cultures.
Location: Boston, MA.
Website: www.unitedplanet.org

Uplift International
Description: A not-for-profit organization, Uplift seeks to deliver emergency relief, humanitarian aid, and health training to improve the well-being of vulnerable populations in Indonesia.
Location: Seattle, WA.
Website: www.upliftinternational.org

Vamos Adelante Foundation
Description: A not-for-profit organization, the foundation provides education, health, and nutrition services to poor people in Guatemala.
Location: Esquintla, Guatemala.
Website: www.vamosadelante.org

Vellore Christian Medical College (CMC) Board (USA)
Description: A not-for-profit organization, the CMC Board supports and promotes Christian Medical College, with medical services and training in Vellore, India.
Location: New York, NY.
Website: www.vellorecmc.org

Vital International Foundation
Description: A not-for-profit organization, the foundation seeks to improve the sexual and reproductive health of people living in Ghana through education and services.

Location: Inglewood, CA.
Website: www.vitalinternational.org

Voluntary Service Overseas (VSO) Canada
Description: A not-for-profit organization, VSO seeks to reduce poverty worldwide.
Location: Ottawa, ON.
Website: www.vsocanada.org

Volunteers for Peace (VFP)
Description: A not-for-profit organization, VFP functions as a placement service for short-term international work projects.
Location: Belmont, VT.
Website: www.vfp.org

Volunteers in Medical Missions (VIMM)
Description: A not-for-profit religiously affiliated organization, VIMM provides opportunities for Christian medical professionals and other volunteers to experience medical missions.
Location: Seneca, SC.
Website: www.vimm.org

World Concern
Description: A not-for-profit organization, World Concern seeks to relieve human suffering and to bring hope and reconciliation by focusing on basic needs, sustainable livelihoods, and family stability.
Location: Seattle, WA.
Website: www.worldconcern.org

World Education
Description: A not-for-profit arm of John Snow Inc., World Education seeks to provide education and opportunities for the socially and economically disadvantaged.
Location: Boston, MA.
Website: www.worlded.org

World Medical Mission (WMM)
Description: A not-for-profit religiously affiliated organization, the WMM offers short- and long-term emergency medical work in Christian hospitals and clinics around the world.

Location: Boone, NC.
Website: www.samaritanspurse.org

World Neighbors
Description: A not-for-profit organization, World Neighbors aims to eliminate hunger, disease, and poverty.
Location: Oklahoma City, OK.
Website: www.wn.org

World University Services Canada (WUSC)
Description: A not-for-profit organization, WUSC seeks to foster human development and global understanding through education and training.
Location: Ottawa, ON.
Website: www.wusc.ca

World Vision
Description: A not-for-profit organization, World Vision provides funding and resources for relief and development projects in developing countries worldwide.
Location: Federal Way, WA.
Website: www.worldvision.org

6 Education in Global Health

Numerous educational opportunities and pathways are available for people interested in learning more about global health and medicine. The more conventional pathways into global health have been through medicine, nursing, public health, and other allied health professions. However, as we have emphasized in earlier chapters, these are certainly not the only paths to a career or experience in global health. Any additional training or educational opportunity that you seek should be related to your interests and motivations in global health, and not by the conventional dogma. For example, if a person is interested in formulating or shaping global health policy, then perhaps a graduate-level degree in foreign affairs would be best. Someone wanting to work with global health economics and financing may find an economics degree to be most appropriate. Similarly, a person interested in infrastructure and land development may want to pursue studies in civil engineering. Virtually any field of study, although some may need some creative thinking, can find an important niche and connection for conducting sustainable work in global health and medicine.

This chapter will focus on educational opportunities for the traditional pathways in global health and medicine. Deciding whether or not to pursue a graduate degree, such as a Master of Public Health, or which graduate degree to pursue are often the most difficult questions. First, deciding not to pursue a graduate degree can be reasonable, but obtaining a position, without sufficient experience, or acquiring more responsibility within a position may prove to be difficult. Nonetheless, one can always choose to return for a graduate degree at any time, and having some experience may help you decide which degree would be most suited to your interests. People primarily interested in providing individual clinical services may be steered towards training as a medical doctor, nurse, or physician's assistant. Those people who are more interested in addressing population-level health and policy issues might be encouraged to consider additional training in public health, foreign affairs, anthropology, health geography, or social work. Deciding whether to obtain a master's or doctoral degree can also be a difficult decision. In general, people working in global health and medicine have varying levels of degrees, and each carries different responsibilities. There is a notion of a 'glass ceiling' for people without a doctoral degree, either a PhD or an MD, but this depends on the organization. In general, an MD often carries a little more credibility and flexibility in global health and medicine than a PhD, but again, this can be dependent on the organization and a person's level of experience.

The most popular degree in global health is a Master of Public Health (MPH). Areas of study that may be included in a public health degree include the following: maternal and child health, population health, family planning, demography, economics, epidemiology and biostatistics, communicable and tropical diseases, public health administration and policy, environmental health, occupational health and safety, nutrition, and health education. For those people who are pursuing or have a medical degree, there is no perfect time to obtain an MPH degree. Obtaining this training before or during medical school may allow for more global health opportunities during training, minimize disruptions, and provide an additional perspective to medical studies. Pursuing an MPH degree after completing the medical degree may provide a longer-term benefit, since it will be fresher and not competing with the loads of medical information. In addition, some medical fellowship programs will often provide the time and funding for their fellows to obtain an MPH degree. One word of advice, however, is to obtain the best training possible for your interests and goals. The reputation of your training institution and the contacts you make at this school can go a long way in boosting your career in global health and medicine.

In the remainder of this chapter, we list contact information for schools of public health around the world with significant global health concentrations. In addition, we provide a listing of established and newly created centres for global health, since they can serve as valuable repositories of information, particularly related to educational opportunities. Finally, we provide a listing of medical residency programs that significantly incorporate global health opportunities into their training programs. We have not included medical schools in this chapter, since most medical schools have now incorporated some degree of global health training opportunities and pathways. Finally, information on educational programs changes often, so be sure to check the websites and contact schools and programs for the most up-to-date details.

Schools of Public Health

There are many schools of public health around the world that adequately address global health issues and topics. The following 31 schools of public health have global health departments or programs and are listed alphabetically by country.

United States

Boston University, School of Public Health, Center for International Health and Development
715 Albany St, Talbot Building, Boston, MA 02118
Phone: (617) 638–4640
Website: sph.bu.edu

Columbia University, Mailman School of Public Health
Office of Admission, 722 West 168th St, Suite 1030, New York, NY 10032
Phone: (212) 342-5127
Website: www.mailman.hs.columbia.edu

Emory Rollins School of Public Health
Grace Crum Rollins Building, 1518 Clifton Rd, Atlanta, GA 30322
Phone: (404) 727-3956
Website: www.sph.emory.edu

George Washington University School of Public Health and Health Sciences
2300 I St NW, Washington, DC 20037
Phone: (202) 994-2160
Website: www.gwumc.edu/sphhs

Harvard School of Public Health
677 Huntington Ave, Boston, MA 02115
Phone: (617) 432-1031
Website: www.hsph.harvard.edu

Johns Hopkins University, Bloomberg School of Public Health
615 N Wolfe St, Baltimore, MD 21205
Phone: (443) 287-7277
Website: www.jhsph.edu

Loma Linda University, School of Public Health
24951 N Circle Dr, Loma Linda, CA 92350
Phone: (909) 558-4694 (Ext. 88036) or (800) 422-4558
Website: www.llu.edu/llu/sph

New York Medical College, School of Public Health
Room 316, Valhalla, NY 10595
Phone: (914) 594-4510
Website: www.nymc.edu/sph

Saint Louis University, School of Public Health
Website: www.slu.edu/colleges/sph/slusph/Default.htm

Tulane University, School of Public Health and Tropical Medicine
1430 Tulane Ave, SL-29, New Orleans, LA 70112
Phone: (504) 988-5388
Website: www.sph.tulane.edu

University of Alabama at Birmingham, School of Public Health
Ryals Public Health Building, 1665 University Bld, Birmingham,
AL 35294-0022
Phone: (205) 934-4993
Website: www.soph.uab.edu

University of California at Berkeley, School of Public Health
140 Warren Hall #7360, Berkeley, CA 94720-7360
Phone: (510) 643-0881
Website: sph.berkeley.edu

University of California at Los Angeles (UCLA), School of Public
Health
16-071 Center for Health Sciences, Box 951772, Los Angeles, CA
90095-1772
Phone: (310) 825-5524
E-mail: info@ph.ucla.edu
Website: www.ph.ucla.edu/admissions_contact.html

University of Michigan, School of Public Health
109 Observatory St, 3537 SPH I, Ann Arbor, MI 48109-2029
Phone: (734) 764-5425
Website: www.sph.umich.edu

University of Minnesota, School of Public Health
420 Delaware St SE, Minneapolis, MN 55455
Phone: (612) 624-6669
Website: www.sph.umn.edu

University of Nebraska, College of Public Health
Phone: (402) 559-4962
Website: www.unmc.edu/publichealth/

University of North Carolina at Chapel Hill, School of Public Health
Website: www.sph.unc.edu

University of Pittsburgh, Graduate School of Public Health
114 Parran Hall, 130 Desoto St, Pittsburgh, PA 15261
Phone: (412) 624-3002
Website: www.publichealth.pitt.edu

University of South Florida, School of Public Health
13201 Bruce B Downs Blvd, MDC 56, Tampa, FL 33612
Phone: (813) 974-3623
Website: publichealth.usf.edu

University of Texas, School of Public Health
PO Box 20186, Houston, TX 77225
Phone: (713) 500-9032
Website: www.sph.uth.tmc.edu

University of Virginia
MR-4 Building, Lane Rd, Room 3146, PO Box 801379, University of
Virginia Health System, Charlottesville, VA 22908-1379
Phone: (434) 924-5242
Website: www.healthsystem.virginia.edu/internet/phs/mph/
mph_home.cfm

University of Washington, School of Public Health and Community
Medicine
International Health Program, Room F-356D, 1959 NE Pacific, Seattle,
WA 98195
Phone: (206) 685-3057
Website: sphcm.washington.edu

Yale University, School of Public Health
47 College St, Suite 108, New Haven, CT 06510
Phone: (203) 785-2844
Website: www.med.yale.edu/eph

Australia

George Institute for International Health
Level 10, King George V Building, Royal Prince Alfred Hospital, Mis-
senden Rd, Camperdown, New South Wales 2050
Phone: 61-2-9993-4500
Website: www.thegeorgeinstitute.org

James Cook University
Department of Health and Tropical Medicine, Townsville, Queensland
4811
Phone: 61-7-4781-4942
Website: www.jcu.edu.au

Brazil

Fundacao Oswaldo Cruz
Website: www.fiocruz.br

Canada

Simon Fraser University
Faculty of Health Sciences
8888 University Dr, Burnaby, BC V5A 1S6
Phone: (604) 268-7036
Website: www.fhs.sfu.ca

University of Alberta School of Public Health
13-103 Clinical Sciences Building, 11350-83 Ave, Edmonton, AB
T6G 2G3
Phone: (780) 492-6682
Website: www.publichealth.ualberta.ca/contact.cfm?nav01=1

University of Ottawa, Population Health
1 Stewart St, Room 300, Ottawa, ON K1N 6N5
Phone: (613) 562-5691
Website: www.grad.uottawa.ca

University of Toronto, Public Health Sciences
155 College St, Room 620, Toronto, ON M5T 3M7
Phone: (416) 978-0901
Website: www.phs.utoronto.ca

Japan

Nagasaki University, Institute of Tropical Medicine
1-12-4, Sakamoto, Nagasaki 752-7523
Website: www.tm.nagasaki-u.ac.jp/english/e-frame.html

Mexico

Instituto Nacional de Salud Publica
Website: www.insp.mx

Switzerland

Swiss Tropical Institute
Socinstrasses 57, PO Box CH-4002, Basel
Website: www.sti.ch

Thailand

Mahidol University, Faculty of Tropical Medicine
420/6 Ratchawithi Rd, Ratchadewee, Bangkok 10400
Phone: 66-0-2354-9100-19
Website: www.mahidol.ac.th

United Kingdom

Liverpool School of Tropical Hygiene and Medicine
Pembroke Place, Liverpool L3 5QA
Phone: 44-151-708-9393
Website: www.liv.ac.uk/lstm/contact/index.htm

London School of Tropical Hygiene and Medicine
Keppel St, London WC1E 7HT
Phone: 44-20-7299-4646
Website: www.lshtm.ac.uk

Centres for Global Health

Several centres for global health have been established and many more
are being planned at academic institutions. Some of these were created
to research specialized areas of global health, but nearly all combine
research and teaching related to global health. These centres for global
health can serve as excellent sources of information for job opportunities or specialized areas of global health training.

United States

Case Western Reserve University, Center for International Health
10900 Euclid Ave, Cleveland, OH 44106-4978
Phone: (216) 368-6321
Website: www.case.edu/orgs/cghd/Home.htm

Harvard Initiative for Global Health
104 Mt Auburn St, 3rd Floor, Cambridge, MA 02138
Phone: (617) 495-8231
Website: www.globalhealth.harvard.edu

Michigan State University, Institute of International Health
Website: www.msu.edu/unit/iih

Mount Sinai School of Medicine
Website: mssm-ghc.org

New York University, School of Medicine
Center for Global Health, Bellevue Hospital, 462 First Ave, NBV 5NEB,
New York, NY 10016

Phone: (212) 263-8118
Website: globalhealth.med.nyu.edu/whoweare/contact.html

Ohio State University, Office of Global Health Education
021 Meiling Hall, 370 West 9th Ave, Columbus, OH 43210
Phone: (614) 247-8968
Website: medicine.osu.edu/globalhealth/1779.cfm

Vanderbilt Institute for Global Health
319 Light Hall, Nashville, TN 37232-0685
Phone: (615) 322-9374
Website: www.mc.vanderbilt.edu/medschool/globalhealth

University of Arizona, College of Medicine
International Health: Clinical and Community Care
Website: www.globalhealth.arizon.edu

University of California at San Francisco, Global Health Sciences and
University of California at Berkeley School of Public Health, Institute
for Global Health
Website: www.globalhealthsciences.ucsf.edu

University of California at San Francisco, Institute for Global Orthope-
dics and Traumatology
Website: www.sfghf.net/docs/IGOT_brochure_v8b_web.pdf

University of Washington, Department of Global Health
Website: depts.washington.edu/deptgh

Wright State University, Center for Global Health Systems, Management and Policy
Website: www.med.wright.edu/hsm/aboutus.html

Canada

Dalhousie University, International Health Office
Website: iho.medicine.dal.ca

McGill University, Global Health Programs
Website: www.mcgill.ca/globalhealth/

University of Alberta
Website: www.international.ualberta.ca

University of British Columbia, Centre for Global Health, Liu Centre
Website: www.cgh.ligi.ubc.ca

University of Calgary, International Health Program
Website: ihp.myweb.med.ucalgary.ca

University of Ottawa, Centre for Global Health
Website: www.intermed.med.uottawa.ca/research/globalhealth/
index.html

University of Toronto, Centre for International Health
Website: intlhealth.med.utoronto.ca/

United Kingdom

University College London, Centre for International Health and
Development
Website: www.ich.ucl.ac.uk/ich/academicunits/cihd/Homepage

Medical Residency Programs

Many medical residency programs offer some time for their residents to
pursue research or international opportunities, particularly towards the
end of the program. In addition to examining the residency program, an
applicant would be wise to look at other non-clinical global health
opportunities at an institution. The degree of support and arrangement
of global health training and international clinical rotations can be
highly variable. The following list includes some of the programs with
significant training or clinical opportunities in global health. This list is
not exhaustive and many programs continue to incorporate global
health training into their curriculum. The programs are listed by medical specialty.

General Residencies

Albert Einstein, Global Health Fellowship
Website: www.aecom.yu.edu/ooe/special_programs/
global_health.htm

Mount Sinai School of Medicine
Website: mssm-ghc.org/electives

University of California at San Francisco
Website: www.globalhealthsciences.ucsf.edu/education/people

Emergency Medicine

Brigham and Women's Hospital (Harvard University), Institute for International Emergency Medicine and Health
Website: www.iemh.org/fellowship.html

Brown University
Website: www.brown.edu/Administration/Emergency_Medicine/emr/pages/IEM_FellowshipMPH.html

Johns Hopkins University, International Emergency Fellowship Program
Website: www.jhsph.edu/Refugee/Education_Training/fellowship

Loma Linda University, International Emergency Fellowship
Website: www.llu.edu/llumc/emergency/international/index.html

Los Angeles County and University of Southern California, Department of Emergency Medicine
Website: www.usc.edu/schools/medicine/departments/emergency_medicine/international/index.html

Medical College of Georgia
Website: www.mcg.edu/ems/residency/International.htm

Rush University Medical Center
Website: www.iemfellowship.org

University of Southern California
LAC + USC Medical Center Department of Emergency Medicine, L 1011, 1200 N State St, Los Angeles, CA 90033
Website: www.usc.edu/schools/medicine/departments/emergency_medicine/international/index.html

Family Medicine

Barberton Family Practice
155 Fifth St NE, Barberton, OH 44203
Phone: (330) 745-5008
Website: www.barbhosp.com

Baylor College of Medicine
5510 Greenbriar Dr, Houston, TX 77005
Phone: (713) 798-7859
Website: www.bcm.edu/familymed/international/index.htm

Carilon Health System
1314 Peters Creek Rd, Roanoke, VA 24017
Phone: (540) 562-5702

Case Western Reserve University, School of Medicine
10900 Euclid Ave, Cleveland, OH 44106
Phone: (216) 844-3791

Chestnut Hill Hospital
8815 Germantown Ave, 5th Floor, Philadelphia, PA 19118
Phone: (215) 248-8145
Website: www.chh.org

Clinton Memorial Hospitals
825 W Locust St, Wilmington, OH 45177
Phone: (937) 383-3382
Website: www.cmhregional.com

Fairfax Family Medicine
Website: www.fairfaxfamilypractice.com/residents.asp

Fairview-University Medical Center
Smiley's Clinic
2615 E Franklin Ave, Minneapolis, MN 55406
Phone: (612) 333-0774
E-mail: residency@famprac.umn.edu

Hennepin County Medical Center
701 Park Ave, Minneapolis, MN 55415

Phone: (612)-873-3000
E-mail: info@hcmc.org

Howard University Hospital
2139 Georgia Ave NW, Suite #3B, Washington, DC 2001
Phone: (202)-865-1452
Website: www.huhosp.org

In His Image Family Practice Residency
7600 S Lewis, Tulsa, OK 74136
Phone: (918) 493-7816
Website: www.inhisimage.org

Jefferson Medical College
1015 Walnut St, Suite 401 C, Philadelphia, PA 19107
Phone: (215) 955-2350
Website: www.tju.edu

Lancaster General Hospital
555 N Duke St, PO Box 3555, Lancaster, PA 17604
Phone: (717) 290-4940

Lutheran Family Practice
6S Lutheran General Hospital, 1775 Dempster St, Park Ridge, IL 60068
Phone: (847) 723-7969
Website: www.lghfpres.com

Madigan Army Medical Center
MCHJ-FP, Tacoma, WA 98431
Phone: (253) 968-1335

Marshall University, School of Medicine
Website: www.meb.marshall.edu/fch

McLennan County Family Practice
1600 Providence Dr, Waco, TX 76707
Phone: (254) 750-8239

Medical College of Georgia, Department of Family Medicine
1120 15th St, Augusta, GA 30912
Phone: (706) 721-3157

Medical College of Wisconsin Columbia St Mary's
8701 Watertown Plan Rd, PO Box 26509, Milwaukee, WI 53226
Phone: (414) 456-4622
Website: www.family.mcw.edu/CSM *or* www.family.mcw.edu/belize

Memorial Hospital
714 N Michigan St, South Bend, IN 46601
Phone: (219) 284-7913
Website: www.qualityoflife.org/fpc.htm

Middlesex Hospital
90 S Main St, Middletown, CT 06457
Phone: (860) 344-6418
Website: www.midhosp.org

Moses H. Cone Memorial Hospital
1125 N Church St, Greensboro, NC 27401
Phone: (336) 832-8132
Website: www.gahec.org/fm

Oregon Health Science University
3181 SW Sam Jackson Park Rd, Portland, OR 97201
Phone: (503) 494-1093

Rush Medical College
Suite 764, Academic Facility, 600 South Paulina St, Chicago, IL 60612
Phone: (773) 296-7151
Website: www.rushu.rush.edu/familymed/stfm

Self Memorial Hospital
160 Academy Ave, Greenwood, SC 29646
Phone: (864) 227-4869

St Elizabeth's Family Practice
1431 North Western Ave, Chicago, IL 60622
Phone: (312) 633-5808
Website: www.stelizabeth.com/services/our_services/fp_residency/

St Joseph's Regional Medical Center
837 E Cedar St, Suite 125, South Bend, IN 46617

Phone: (574) 237-7637
Website: www.sjmed.com

St Luke's Family Practice Residency
2801 W Kinnickinnic River Pkwy, Suite 175, Milwaukee, WI 53215
Phone: (414) 649-7909
Website: www.aurorahealthcare.com

St Mary's
3700 Washington Ave, Evansville, IN 47750
Phone: (812) 485-4173
Website: www.stmarys.org

St Vincent Family Medicine Residency Program
8220 Naab Rd, Suite 200, Indianapolis, IN 46260
Phone: (317) 338-7600
Website: www.stvincent.org

Tallahassee Memorial HealthCare
1301 Hodges Dr, Tallahassee, FL 32308
Phone: (850) 431-5714
Website: tmh.org

University of Arizona
Family Practice Residency Program, Tucson, Arizona
Phone: (520) 694-1607
Website: www.fem.arizona.edu/residency

University of California at Irvine
101 The City Dr S, Bldg 200, Rt 81, Orange, CA 92868
Phone: (714) 456-5171
Website: www.ucihs.uci.edu

University of California at Los Angeles, School of Medicine
10833 Le Conte Ave, Los Angeles, CA 90095
Phone: (310) 825-8234

University of Cincinnati – Mercy Franciscan Hospital, Family Medicine
Residency Program
Christ Hospital, 2139 Auburn Ave, Cincinnati, OH 45219

Phone: (513) 585-2000
Website: www.familymedicine.uc.edu/residency/international/
internationalhome.htm

University of Florida
Box 103588, Gainesville, FL 32610
Phone: (352) 392-4541

University of Hawaii
95-390 Kuahelani St, Honolulu, HI 96789
Phone: (808) 627-3247

University of Iowa
200 Hawkins Dr, Iowa City, IA 52242
Phone: (319) 384-7500

University of Kansas at Wichita, School of Medicine
1010 N Kansas St, Wichita, KS 67214
Phone: (316) 293-2607
Website: wichita.kumc.edu/fcm

University of Massachusetts
55 Lake Ave N, Worcester, MA 01655
Phone: (508) 856-3914
Website: www.umassmed.edu

University of Michigan
L2003 Womens–Box 0239, Ann Arbor, MI 48109
Phone: (734) 615-2688
Website: www.med.umich.edu/fammed/

University of Minnesota, St John's Hospital
1414 Maryland Ave E, St Paul, MN 55106
Phone: (651) 772-3461
Website: www.med.umn.edu

University of Minnesota, St Joseph's Hospital, Family Medicine
Residency Program
Website: www.med.umn.edu/fm/residency/stjosephs/home.html

University of Mississippi, Department of Family Medicine
2500 N State St, Jackson, MS 39216
Phone: (601) 984-5426

University of Nebraska Medical Center
Omaha, Nebraska
Website: app1.unmc.edu/fammed/

University of New Mexico, Health Sciences Center
Family Practice Center, 3rd Floor, 2400 Tucker Ave NE, Albuquerque,
NM 87131
Phone: (505) 272-2165

University of Oklahoma at Tulsa, CS Lewis Jr, College of Medicine
9920 East 21st St, Tulsa, OK 74129
Phone: (918) 838-4752
Website: www.tulsa.ouhsc.edu

University of Rochester, Medical Center
Website: www.urmc.rochester.edu/fammed/iht/overseas_sites.cfm

University of Tennessee at Knoxville, Department of Family Medicine
1924 Alcoa Highway, Knoxville, TN 37920
Phone: (865) 544-9352
Website: gsm.utmck.edu/mrc/main.htm

University of Tennessee at Memphis, College of Medicine
1127 Union Ave, Memphis, TN 38104
Phone: (901) 448-5216
Website: www.utmem.edu/fammed

University of Utah, School of Medicine
50 N Medical Dr, Salt Lake City, UT 84132
Phone: (801) 581-7766
Website: www.utah.edu/upap

University of Wyoming
821 East 18th St, Cheyenne, WY 82001
Phone: (307) 777-7911
Website: www.uwyo.edu/chyfamprac

Valley Baptist Medical Center
2222 Benwood St, Harlingen, TX 78550
Phone: (956) 389-2248
Website: www.vbfpr.com

Internal Medicine

Baylor College of Medicine, Department of International Medicine
One Baylor Plaza, Houston, TX, 77030
Phone: (800)-553-9559
Website: www.bcm.edu/medicine/residency/?PMID=3953

Brigham and Women's Hospital
Website: www.brighamandwomens.org/socialmedicine/ghecontacts.
aspx

Brown University
Website: www.brownmedicine.org/education/international.asp?
section=education

Columbia University
Website: www.columbiamedicine.org/education/r_apply.shtml

Dartmouth University, Dartmouth-Hitchcock Medical Center
One Medical Centre Dr, Lebanon, NH 03756
Website: www.dhmc.org/webpage.cfm?site_id=2&org_id=33&gsec_id
=0&sec_id=0&i tem_id=1095

Duke University
Website: medicine.duke.edu/modules/fellowship/index.php?id=3

Emory University
Website: medicine.emory.edu/residency/contactus.cfm

Indiana University
1001 West 10th St, WD OPW M200, Indianapolis, IN 46202
Website: medicine.iupui.edu/residency

Johns Hopkins University
2024 E Monument St, Suite 2-600, Baltimore, MD 21205
Website: www.hopkinsmedicine.org/gim/fellowship/index.html

Massachusetts General Hospital (part of Harvard Medical School)
55 Fruit St, Boston, MA 02114
Website: www.massgeneral.org/medicine/index.asp?page=residency

Mount Sinai Hospital
One Gustave L Levy Place, Box 1118, New York, NY 10029
Website: www.mssm.edu/medicine/residency/apply.shtml

Tulane University
Website: www.som.tulane.edu/departments/medicine

University of California at Davis
Website: www.ucdmc.ucdavis.edu/internalmedicine/residency.html

University of California at Los Angeles, UCLA Medical Center, Department of Medicine
Los Angeles, CA 90095-1736
Website: www.imresidency.med.ucla.edu

University of California at San Francisco
Website: medicine.ucsf.edu/residency/overview

University of Colorado
4200 East 9th Ave, B177, Denver, CO 80262
Website: www.uchsc.edu/sm/intmed/main/contact.php

University of Miami (Jay Weiss Residency)
1500 NW 12th Ave, Suite 1020-E, Miami, FL 33136
Website: www.jayweisscenter.org/x14.xml

University of Minnesota
Website: www.globalhealth.umn.edu

University of Pennsylvania
Website: residency.dom.pitt.edu/Program_Overview/tracks/globalhealth.html

University of Pittsburgh, Global Health Track
UPMC Montefiore Hospital, Suite 933W, 200 Lothrop St, Pittsburgh, PA 15213
Website: residency.dom.pitt.edu/Program_Overview/tracks/globalhealth.html

University of Virginia
Internal Medicine Residency Recruitment Office, PO Box 800696,
University of Virginia Health System, Charlottesville, VA 22908
Website: www.healthsystem.virginia.edu/internet/im-residapp/
apply.cfm

University of Washington
Website: depts.washington.edu/uwmedres/

West Virginia University
Website: www.health.wvu.edu/international/index.html

Yale University, Internal Medicine/Primary Care
Website: www.med.yale.edu/intmed/genmed/pages/barry.html

Pediatrics

Brown University
Website: www.brown.edu/Departments/Pediatrics/Residency/
Homepage/redesign/index.html

Case Western Reserve University, Center for Global Child Health
11000 Euclid Ave, Mailstop – TBC6008, Cleveland, OH 44106
Phone: (216) 844-8918
Website: www.uhhospitals.org/rainbowchildren/tabid/689/
Default.aspx

Children's Hospital of Philadelphia, Graduate Medical Education
Phone: 215-590-2437
Website: www.chop.edu/consumer/jsp/microsite/microsite.jsp?id
=81643

Emory University
49 Jesse Hill Jr Dr SE, Atlanta, GA 30303
Phone: (404) 778-1401
Website: www.pediatrics.emory.edu/residency/fellowships1.htm

University of California at San Francisco
Box 0110, M-691, San Francisco, CA 94143-0110

Phone: (415)-476-5001
Website: www.pediatrics.medschool.ucsf.edu/brochure

University of Minnesota, Pediatric Global Health Track
Pediatric Infectious Diseases
420 Delaware St, SE, MMC 296, Minneapolis, MN 55455
Phone: (612) 624-1112
Website: www.med.umn.edu/peds/globalpediatrics/home.html

University of Washington
4800 Sand Point Way NE, PO Box 5371/G-0061, Seattle, WA 98105-0371
Phone: (206)-987-5080
Website: uwpeds.seattlechildrens.org/apply

Plastic Surgery

Loma Linda University
Website: www.llu.edu/llu/medicine/plastics/outreach.htm

Surgery

Brown University
Phone: (401) 444-5180
Website: bms.brown.edu/surgery/pages/program.html

Mount Sinai School of Medicine
Website: www.mssm.edu/surgery/residency/overseas.shtml

7 Funding for Global Health Opportunities

'But how will I pay for it?' is the often asked question regarding a global health experience abroad. There are myriad possibilities for funding an adventure in global health. This chapter explores different possibilities for financing global health journeys and includes websites for specific grants, scholarships, fellowships, and other funding sources that may help make a global health experience possible and affordable.

For a health profession student, financial aid comes in three basic forms: governmental (state and federal aid), institutional (funded by the student's college or university), and private (typically funded by various civic, religious, and professional organizations).

U.S. Governmental Aid

Aid (including federally funded loans) may be available from the U.S. government through the institution where the student is enrolled. Restrictions regarding governmental aid vary by institution, and interested students should consult with the campus study abroad adviser or financial aid counsellor to determine eligibility. A student who currently receives federal financial aid and has completed the Federal Application for Federal Student Aid (FAFSA) form for the academic year in which study abroad is planned will not need to resubmit the form. A student who has not previously submitted a FAFSA should allow plenty of time to do so. There are also a variety of foreign institutions that offer financial aid independently of any U.S. institution. Currently 503 such institutions and their federal school codes can be found on the U.S. government's website 'Federal Application for Federal Student Aid' (www.fafsa.edu/gov).

Institutional Aid

Financial assistance may be offered by the student's college or university for students enrolled at that institution. The study abroad office or its website is often the best source for identifying such funding, which may be in the form of scholarships, grants, or fellowships. Institutional aid may or may not be used to finance study abroad, depending on any restrictions associated with the award.

Private Aid

Private aid includes funds from non-governmental, non-institutional sources and may also be available to individuals not currently enrolled in an academic program. Sources for private aid include the following:

- Foundations
- Religious organizations
- Civic and service groups
- Professional organizations (especially local and state chapters)
- Ethnic groups
- Special interest clubs
- Alumni associations
- Charitable organizations
- Sororities and fraternities (local and national chapters)
- Local and regional corporations
- Sister City chapters
- Partners of the America local chapters

These organizations may offer funding for specific global health programs or may be receptive to specific, unsolicited fundraising proposals. In addition, family and friends may also be significant sources of private aid.

Ideas for Creative Fundraising

If you don't have governmental, institutional, or private financial assistance secured for your global health experience or if the funding doesn't fully fund your experience, then you may wish to engage in personal fundraising. Not only will fundraising make your global health experience more affordable, but it can also serve as an educational forum to raise global health awareness.

Carefully prepared, direct proposals are best. Your request should include an anticipated budget that identifies the gains for the funding organization, the host country and institution, and for you. An appeal that reflects enthusiasm, creativity, and sincerity will enhance your chances of success. Perseverance is often a necessary component of the funding process, so don't fear a rejection or take it personally.

Let the proposed donors know what you will do for them in exchange for their support. Possibilities include:

- Providing regular updates while abroad
- Giving a formal presentation upon return
- Creating a website
- Organizing a discussion
- Organizing a campus or community forum
- Participating in community service or outreach
- Assisting others in arranging similar experiences

Careful attention to follow-up not only allows the donor group to see the results of its financial support, but lays the groundwork for future solicitation.

Student groups and individuals have utilized many creative and unique approaches to fundraising for global health projects. Keep in mind that your energy and enthusiasm for a global health experience is contagious! A few more ideas for creative fundraising include the following:

- Silent and live auctions
- Selling T-shirts and other clothing items
- Selling fairly traded coffee, chocolate, etc.
- Car washes
- Bake sales
- Concerts
- Raffles
- Concession sales

Existing Sources for Global Health Funding

Health Profession Students

Advanced Study or Research in Scandinavia
Sponsor: American-Scandinavian Foundation.
Target applicant: A U.S. citizen or permanent resident who has completed undergraduate education.
Location: Denmark, Finland, Iceland, Norway, or Sweden.
Description: Applicants must have a well-defined research or study project that makes a stay in Scandinavia essential. Awards are made in all fields.
Stipend: Awards support project-related costs, including maintenance and travel. Fellowships awards (for year-long study) are up to $20,000 and grants (for 1 to 3 months of study) are normally $4,000.
Website: www.amscan.org

Allied Epidemiology Fellowship
Sponsor: Centers for Disease Control Foundation.
Target applicant: A medical student completing the second or third year of medical school.
Location: Centers for Disease Control and Prevention in Atlanta, Georgia.
Description: One year provides students with an applied hands-on training experience in epidemiology and public health.
Stipend: Living expenses covered.
Website: www.cdcfoundation.org

AMSA Global AIDS Fellowship Application
Sponsor: American Medical Student Association.
Target applicant: A U.S. medical student.
Location: Reston, Virginia.
Description: The Global AIDS Fellowship will enable the recipient to utilize the health professions and health students to address the global HIV/AIDS pandemic through education, service, and action, reflecting the need to eliminate global health disparities. Duration of the fellowship is 13 months.
Stipend: 85% of PGY-1 salary.
Website: www.amsa.org

AMSA Global Health Scholars Program
Sponsor: American Medical Students Association.
Target applicant: A health professional student with a focused interest in global health issues; must be member of AMSA.
Location: U.S. institution.
Description: The 8-month program allows promising, motivated students to develop advanced advocacy, communication, and critical thinking skills with which to effect change in global health. The program is carried out over and above the student's academic curriculum.
Stipend: Scholars will be eligible for financial support after four of the six requirements are met.
Website: www.amsa.org

AMWA Overseas Assistance Grant
Sponsor: American Medical Women's Association/American Women's Hospitals Service.
Target applicant: A national AMWA student or resident member. Medical students must be completing their second, third, or fourth year at an accredited U.S. medical school.
Location: Off-campus setting where the medically neglected will benefit.
Description: Six weeks to 1 year will be spent in a sponsored program that will serve the needs of the medically underserved.
Stipend: Up to $1,500.
Website: www.amwa-doc.org

AWC Scholarship
Sponsor: American Women's Club in Stockholm (AWC).
Target applicant: A U.S. female citizen, 18 years or older, currently living in the United States.
Location: Sweden.
Description: The AWC makes it possible for American women to study in Sweden. The scholarship is awarded for academic excellence. The applicant must be accepted for a period of study or research at a Swedish educational institute. All academic fields are eligible.
Stipend: $1,500 travel grant.
Website: www.awcstockholm.org

Benjamin H. Kean Traveling Fellowship in Tropical Medicine
Sponsor: American Society of Tropical Medicine and Hygiene (ASTMH).

Target applicant: A North American full-time medical student interested in tropical medicine and global health. Preference will be given to applicants sponsored by a member of the ASTMH Clinical Group.
Location: Tropical location.
Description: This is a clinical or research elective in the tropics of at least 1-month duration.
Stipend: Up to $700 towards living expenses and round-trip airfare.
Website: www.astmh.org

Charles S. Houston Research Award
Sponsor: Wilderness Medicine Society.
Target applicant: A medical student.
Location: Not specified.
Description: Award recipients will conduct well-defined projects likely to result in a substantive contribution to the field of wilderness medicine.
Stipend: Up to $5,000.
Website: www.wms.org

Doris Duke International Clinical Research Fellowship
Sponsor: Doris Duke Charitable Foundation.
Target applicant: A student attending a U.S. medical school who has completed 2 or more years of medical school.
Location: Africa.
Description: A 1-year fellowship, 8 months of which will be spent conducting HIV/AIDS and related diseases research in Africa.
Stipend: $27,000 stipend, health insurance, financial support to attend research meetings, and supplementary research and training funds.
Website: www.ddcf.org

Fulbright Program for U.S. Students
Sponsor: U.S. Department of State.
Target applicant: A graduating senior, recent graduate, or graduate student; must be a U.S. citizen at the time of application.
Location: Many countries around the world.
Description: Fellowships are awarded for study, research, internships and/or service abroad (approximately 1,200 awards per year).
Stipend: Full grants include airfare, maintenance for the academic year, book and research allowances, and miscellaneous costs.
Website: us.fulbrightonline.org

GHM Travel Assistance Grants
Sponsor: Global Health Ministries (GHM).
Target applicant: A Lutheran medical or dental student.
Location: Overseas Lutheran hospitals.
Description: GHM provides travel assistance grants to Lutheran medi-cal/dental students who spend one quarter in an overseas Lutheran Hospital.
Stipend: $1,000.
Website: www.ghm.org

Global Health Council Internship Program
Sponsor: Global Health Council (GHC).
Target applicant: A graduate or undergraduate student at an accredited university.
Location: Washington, DC, or White River Junction, Vermont.
Description: The GHC internships offer students unique learning experiences in advocating and supporting programs that improve health around the world; 30 hours per week over 12 weeks.
Stipend: $200 per month.
Website: www.globalhealth.org

Global Health Fellows
Sponsor: U.S. Agency for International Development (USAID).
Target applicant: An outstanding student or mid-career changer interested in pursuing a career in international development.
Location: Washington, DC.
Description: Ten-week summer internships at USAID's Bureau for Global Health in various areas.
Stipend: Hourly rate based on education and experience.
Website: www.ghfp.net

HHMI Research Training Fellowships for Medical and Dental Students
Sponsor: Howard Hughes Medical Institute (HHMI).
Target applicant: A medical or dental student currently enrolled in a U.S. institution.
Location: Arranged with the academic institutions; can be international.
Description: The HHMI Fellowships provide support for 1 year of full-time research training in fundamental biomedical research. The research must be conducted at an academic or non-profit research institution in the United States, excluding the NIH. Research may be con-

ducted at an institution outside the United States as long as the fellow's mentor is affiliated with the U.S. fellowship institution. The fellowship institution need not be the student's medical or dental school.
Stipend: $25,000 for the fellowship year. Fellowship institutions receive annually on behalf of each fellow $5,500 in research allowance and $5,500 allowance to be used for health insurance, tuition, registration fees, etc.
Website: www.hhmi.org

HIVCorps
Sponsor: Centre for Infectious Disease Research in Zambia (CIDRZ)
Target applicant: A pre-medical or pre-M.P.H. student (including one graduating from a post-baccalaureate program), a medical or nursing student, or a recent M.P.H. graduate who wishes to gain international experience.
Location: Zambia.
Description: This 10- to 12-month program is designed to provide students and recent graduates with the opportunity to participate in international HIV programs and research initiatives.
Stipend: Monthly stipend of $1,000, to cover basic living expenses and airfare to Zambia. Housing, costs related to program activities, and local and emergency evacuation insurance is also provided.
Website: www.cirdz.org

India Elective Travel Scholarship
Sponsor: American Association of Physicians of Indian Origin (AAPI).
Target applicant: A student, resident, or fellow in an accredited U.S. scholar training program; must be a member of the AAPI medical student, resident, and fellows section.
Location: India.
Description: The scholarship provides three scholarships to subsidize educational electives in India.
Stipend: $1,000.
Website: www.aapimsr.org

James S. Westra Memorial Endowment Fund
Sponsor: Christian Medical and Dental Associations (CMDA).
Target applicant: A third- or fourth-year medical or dental student enrolled in a traditional program in an approved medical or dental school; must be a CMDA member.

Location: Developing countries.
Description: The fund provides selected medical and dental students with clinical experiences in mission settings that will enable them to become familiar with the cultural, social, and medical problems in developing countries while allowing them to serve the underserved.
Stipend: Up to $500.
Website: www.cmdahome.org

Lambaréné Schweitzer Fellowship
Sponsor: Albert Schweitzer Fellowship.
Target applicant: A senior medical student who is attending a school in New England or New York, or a school elsewhere that participates in the U.S. Schweitzer Fellow Program. Fluency in French is required.
Location: Albert Schweitzer Hospital in Lambaréné, Gabon.
Description: Three-month clinical rotations in pediatrics or medicine.
Stipend: Complete funding (airfare, room, board, immunizations, etc.).
Website: www.schweitzerfellowship.org

Luce Scholars Program
Sponsor: Henry Luce Foundation.
Target applicant: The candidates must be American citizens who have received at least a bachelor's degree and are no more than 29 years old. Those who have significant experience in Asia or Asian studies are not eligible for the program. Nominees must have a record of high achievement, outstanding leadership ability, and a clearly defined career interest with evidence of potential for professional accomplishment.
Location: Asia.
Description: The Luce Scholars Program provides stipends and internships for 18 Americans to live and work in Asia each year. Placement and support services are provided by the Asia Foundation. Sixty-seven U.S. colleges and universities are eligible to make nominations for the program.
Stipend: Basic stipend plus cost-of-living allowance and basic housing allowance where necessary.
Website: www.hluce.org

MAP International Medical Fellowship
Sponsor: Medical Assistance Programs (MAP).
Target applicant: A third- or fourth-year medical student, resident, or intern.

Location: Mission agency or hospital that has an outreach among the poor in a rural or urban setting.
Description: MAP provides exposure in a Christian context to the health, social, and cultural characteristics of a developing community. Students must spend at least 8 weeks in the field; 6 weeks for residents and interns.
Stipend: Round-trip airfare to destination.
Website: www.map.org

O.C. Hubert Student Fellowship in International Health
Sponsor: Centers for Disease Control (CDC) Foundation.
Target applicant: A third- or fourth-year medical or veterinary student.
Location: Developing countries.
Description: Work is to be on a priority health problem in a developing country in conjunction with CDC staff.
Stipend: $3,000 to cover travel costs.
Website: www.cdcfoundation.org

Reproductive Health Externship (RHE) Program
Sponsor: Medical Students for Choice.
Target applicant: A currently enrolled medical student in the United States or Canada.
Location: United States or Canada; other sites possible.
Description: The goal of the RHE is to support students' efforts to obtain clinical exposure to abortion care.
Stipend: Up to $1,000.
Website: www.ms4c.org

Rotary Ambassadorial Scholarship
Sponsor: Rotary International.
Target applicant: Anyone with at least 2 years of college or vocational study.
Location: Open.
Description: The Ambassadorial Scholarships program furthers international understanding and friendly relations among people of different countries. Academic-year and multiyear scholarships are available. Medical internships or residencies are not allowed. Scholars in medical studies during the scholarship period are not permitted to engage in hands-on procedures or direct-care patient services.
Stipend: Academic-year scholarships provide a flat grant of $23,000 for

1 academic year of study in another country. This award is intended to help defray costs of round-trip transportation, tuition, fees, room and board expenses, and miscellaneous expenses. Multiyear scholarships are for 2 years of degree-oriented study in another country. A flat grant of $11,500 is provided per year to be applied towards the costs of a degree program.
Website: www.rotary.org

Sara's Wish Scholarship Fund
Sponsor: Sara's Wish Foundation.
Target applicant: An extraordinary young woman committed to making the world a better place by fully participating in it.
Location: All areas of the globe.
Description: Sara Christie Schewe was killed in her junior year at college in a bus crash in India while participating in the Semester at Sea Program. Sara's Wish Foundation educational travel scholarships are awarded to young women who perpetuate Sara's ideals.
Stipend: TBD. Previous awardees have received between $1,000 and $1,500.
Website: www.saraswish.org

Service Learning Program (SLP) in China
Sponsor: Wang Foundation.
Target applicant: A U.S. student from any major and at any level of undergraduate or graduate study.
Location: China.
Description: The primary task of SLP participants is teaching conversational English to local teachers and public officials in 22 of China's provinces. At the same time, the program helps U.S. participants learn first-hand about the real China by delivering community services on a personal level. U.S. students also have the opportunity to conduct research in areas of their academic interest. The SLP includes 1 week of orientation in Beijing, followed by 4 weeks residing and working in the assigned site.
Stipend: In-country costs are offset by Wang Foundation scholarships awarded to all participants admitted into the program. The scholarship covers room and board expenses incurred inside China, including the week of orientation in Beijing and the 4 weeks at the service site, plus public ground transportation to and from the service site.
Website: www.wangfoundation.net

Shine-a-light Fellowship
Sponsor: Shine-a-light.
Target applicant: A graduate student in medicine, psychology, or another field that can help agencies working with street kids.
Location: Latin America.
Description: Three-month fellowship to work with street children.
Stipend: $1,500 for airfare and housing.
Website: www.shinealight.org/fellowships.html

William B. Bean Student Research Award
Sponsor: American Osler Society.
Target applicant: A currently matriculated student in an approved school of medicine in the United States or Canada.
Location: Open.
Description: The research award supports research in the broad areas of medical history and medical humanism.
Stipend: $1,500 and up to $750 additional may be available to support travel to the society's annual meeting.
Website: americanosler.org

Graduate Students

AAUW International Fellowships
Sponsor: American Association of University Women.
Target applicant: A woman who is a U.S. citizen or permanent resident for graduate or post-graduate study.
Location: Any country, other than the recipient's own.
Description: Fellowships are awarded for full-time study or research. Home Country Project Grants support community-based projects designed to improve the lives of women and girls in the fellow's home country.
Stipend: $18,000 to $30,000 for a fellowship; $5,000 to $7,000 for Home Country Project Grants.
Website: www.aauw.org

Advanced Study or Research in Scandinavia
Sponsor: American-Scandinavian Foundation.
Target applicant: A U.S. citizen or permanent resident who has completed undergraduate education.
Location: Denmark, Finland, Iceland, Norway, or Sweden.

Description: Applicants must have a well-defined research or study project that makes a stay in Scandinavia essential. Awards are made in all fields.
Stipend: Awards support project-related costs, including maintenance and travel. Fellowships awards (for year-long study) are up to $20,000 and grants (for 1 to 3 months of study) are normally $4,000.
Website: www.amscan.org

APHA International Health Scholarships
Sponsor: Colgate Palmolive and the American Public Health Association.
Target applicant: A faculty member or student in a school of public health.
Location: Preference given to select countries.
Description: Grants awarded for community-based projects investigating the role of hygiene in personal and community health and infection control.
Stipend: $10,000 to $15,000.
Website: www.apha-ih.org

AWC Scholarship
Sponsor: American Women's Club in Stockholm (AWC).
Target applicant: A U.S. female citizen, 18 years or older, currently living in the United States.
Location: Sweden.
Description: The AWC makes it possible for American women to study in Sweden. The scholarship is awarded for academic excellence. The applicant must be accepted for a period of study or research at a Swedish educational institution. All academic fields are eligible.
Stipend: $1,500 travel grant.
Website: www.awcstockholm.org

BAEF Fellowship for Study and Research in Belgium
Sponsor: Belgian American Educational Foundation (BAEF).
Target applicant: A U.S. citizen with a master's degree or studying towards a PhD or equivalent degree, with preference given to an applicant under the age of 30 who has a reading and speaking knowledge of Dutch, French, or German.
Location: Belgium.
Description: The program encourages advanced study or research at a Belgian university or institution of higher learning.

Stipend: $21,000 for 1 year of study.
Website: www.baef.be

Chateaubriand Fellowship
Sponsor: Embassy of France in the United States.
Target applicant: A doctoral student enrolled in a U.S. university (cannot be a French citizen).
Location: France.
Description: The Chateaubriand Fellowship allows doctoral students to benefit from an experience to conduct research in France for 9 months.
Stipend: Approximately 1,300 Euros per month, a round-trip ticket to France, health insurance, and 30 Euros per diem for travelling in France for research purposes.
Website: www.france-science.org

Christine Mirzayan Science and Technology Policy Graduate Fellowship Program
Sponsor: National Academies.
Target applicant: A current graduate student or postdoc or scholar who has completed graduate studies or post-doctoral research within the past 5 years in any of the following fields: a physical, biological, or social science or any field of engineering, medicine or health, or veterinary medicine, as well as business, law, education, and other professional programs.
Location: Washington, DC.
Description: The program is designed to engage graduate science, engineering, medical, veterinary, business, and law students in the analysis that informs the creation of science and technology, and government.
Stipend: $5,300 for the 10-week program.
Website: www7.nationalacademies.org

Exploration Fund
Sponsor: Explorers Club.
Target applicant: A graduate student or young scientist.
Location: Not specified.
Description: Grants are awarded to graduate students and young scientists in support of exploration and field research for those who are beginning their research careers.
Stipend: $500 to $1,500
Website: www.explorers.org

Ford Foundation International Fellowship Program (IFP)
Sponsor: Ford Foundation.
Target applicant: A resident national of an eligible IFP country or territory (does not include the United States).
Location: In the applicant's country of origin.
Description: The IFP was developed to provide opportunities for advanced study to exceptional individuals who will use this education to become leaders in their respective fields, furthering development in their own countries and greater economic and social justice worldwide.
Stipend: Financial assistance for travel, living expenses, tuition and related costs, and training costs as required.
Website: www.fordifp.net

Fulbright Program for U.S. Students
Sponsor: U.S. Department of State.
Target applicant: A graduating senior, recent graduate, or graduate student; must be a U.S. citizen at the time of application.
Location: Many countries.
Description: Fellowships are awarded for study, research, internships, and/or service abroad (approximately 1,200 awards per year).
Stipend: Full grants include airfare, maintenance for the academic year, book and research allowances, and miscellaneous costs.
Website: us.fulbrightonline.org

Global Health Council Internship Program
Sponsor: Global Health Council.
Target applicant: A graduate or undergraduate student at an accredited university.
Location: Washington, DC, or White River Junction, Vermont.
Description: The GHC internships offer students unique learning experiences in advocating and supporting programs that improve health around the world; 30 hours per week over 12 weeks.
Stipend: $200 per month.
Website: www.globalhealth.org

Global Health Fellows
Sponsor: U.S. Agency for International Development (USAID).
Target applicant: An outstanding student or mid-career changer interested in pursuing a career in international development.
Location: Washington, DC.

Description: Ten-week summer internships at USAID's Bureau for Global Health in various areas.
Stipend: Hourly rate based on education and experience.
Website: www.ghfp.net

Guggenheim Foundation Dissertation Fellowship
Sponsor: Harry Frank Guggenheim Foundation.
Target applicant: A doctoral candidate who is a citizen of any country, studying at a college in any country.
Location: Unspecified.
Description: The foundation awards fellowships designed to contribute to the support of the doctoral candidate to enable thesis completion within the award year. Research in the natural and social sciences and the humanities studying causes, manifestations, and control of violence, aggression, and dominance is welcomed.
Stipend: $15,000.
Website: www.hfg.org

HIVCorps
Sponsor: Centre for Infectious Diseases Research in Zambia (CIDRZ).
Target applicant: A pre-medical or pre-M.P.H. student (including one graduating from a post-baccalaureate program), a medical or nursing student, or recent M.P.H. graduate who wishes to gain international experience.
Location: Zambia.
Description: This 10- to 12-month program is designed to provide students and recent graduates with the opportunity to participate in international HIV programs and research initiatives.
Stipend: Monthly stipend of $1,000, to cover basic living expenses and airfare to Zambia. Housing, costs related to program activities, and local and emergency evacuation insurance is also provided.
Website: www.hopkinsglobalhealth.org/resources/funding/HIVCorps.pdf

IFUW International Awards
Sponsor: International Federation of University Women (IFUW).
Target applicant: A woman graduate who is a member of an IFUW national federation and association or an IFUW international member.
Location: Any country other than the one in which the applicant was educated or habitually resides.

Description: Fellowships, 8 to 12 months long, are offered for the second and subsequent years of a doctoral program and for post-doctoral studies. Grants are for a minimum of 2 months of work.
Stipend: Based on the award.
Website: www.ifuw.org

International Scholarship Programme
Sponsor: Aga Khan Foundation.
Target applicant: A post-graduate student from a developing country who has no other means of financing her or his studies.
Location: Unspecified.
Description: The Aga Khan Foundation provides a limited number of scholarships to outstanding students from developing countries. Applicants are expected to have some years of work experience in their field of interest. Preference is given to students under 30 years of age.
Stipend: The scholarships are 50% grant, 50% loan, and they assist with tuition and living expenses.
Website: www.akdn.org

JSPS Fellowships
Sponsor: Japan Society for the Promotion of Science (JSPS).
Target applicant: A doctoral student or researcher who is a United Kingdom national and is studying or has graduated from a U.K. institution and is currently conducting research at that institution.
Location: Japan.
Description: The program allows applicants to conduct research with Japanese colleagues in a designated area. A variety of short- and long-term fellowships are available.
Stipend: Airfare, maintenance allowance, and domestic research travel allowance, with additional support provided for longer-term positions.
Website: www.jsps.org

Luce Scholars Program
Sponsor: Henry Luce Foundation.
Target applicant: The candidate must be a U.S. citizen who has received at least a bachelor's degree and is no more than 29 years old. Those who have significant experience in Asia or Asian studies are not eligible for the program. Nominees must have a record of high achievement, outstanding leadership ability, and a clearly defined career interest with evidence of potential for professional accomplishment.

Location: Asia.
Description: The Luce Scholars Program provides stipends and internships for 18 Americans to live and work in Asia each year. Placement and support services are provided by the Asia Foundation. Sixty-seven U.S. colleges and universities are eligible to make nominations for the program.
Stipend: Basic stipend plus cost-of-living allowance and basic housing allowance where necessary.
Website: www.hluce.org

NEW AID Scholarship
Sponsor: NEW AID Foundation
Target applicant: A public health graduate student or a scientist early in her or his career.
Location: Latin America, Asia, Africa, or Eastern Europe. Other areas evaluated on a case-by-case basis.
Description: Stipends are awarded to conduct public health research abroad of the abandoned infectious diseases of marginalized populations.
Stipend: Up to $4,500.
Website: www.newaid.org

Norwegian Thanksgiving Fund Scholarship
Sponsor: American Scandinavian Foundation.
Target applicant: A U.S. citizen who is doing graduate-level work.
Location: Norwegian university.
Description: This award provides assistance for graduate-level work in Norway. Various academic areas are supported, including social medicine.
Stipend: Up to $3,000.
Website: www.amscan.org

NSEP David L. Boren Graduate Fellowships
Sponsor: National Security Education Program.
Target applicant: A U.S. citizen who is applying to or is enrolled in a graduate degree program at an accredited U.S. college or university located in the United States.
Location: World regions that are critical to U.S. interest (including Africa, Asia, Central and Eastern Europe, Eurasia, Latin America and the Caribbean, and the Middle East).

Description: The NSEP Boren Fellowships support students pursuing the study of languages, cultures, regions, and topics that are deemed critical to U.S. national security. This encompasses traditional concerns, as well as challenges of global society, including: sustainable development, environmental degradation, global disease and hunger, population growth and migration, and economic competitiveness. The fellowships include an NSEP service requirement. Fellowship duration is from one semester to 2 academic years.
Stipend: Maximum support is $30,000.
Website: www.iie.org/programs/nsep

SDE/GWIS Fellowships
Sponsor: Sigma Delta Epsilon (SDE) and Graduate Women in Science (GWIS).
Target applicant: An SDE/GWIS member who is enrolled as a graduate student or engaged in post-doctoral or early-stage junior faculty academic research and who has demonstrated financial need.
Location: Unspecified.
Description: The SDE/GWIS Fellowships are academic year awards that can be used for applied or basic research. The overall purpose is to increase the fundamental knowledge of the sciences, and increase the visibility of women with careers in scientific research.
Stipend: Based on the award category, up to $4,000.
Website: www.gwis.org

TWOWS Post-graduate Training Fellowships
Sponsor: Third World Organization for Women in Science (TWOWS).
Target applicant: A female student in sub-Saharan Africa or in a least-developed country who wishes to pursue post-graduate training leading to a doctoral degree.
Location: Developing countries.
Description: The TWOWS Fellowship program contributes to the emergence of a new generation of women leaders in science and technology, and to promote their effective participation in the scientific and technological development of their countries. Each fellowship will be offered for a maximum of 3 years.
Stipend: Monthly living allowance and travel expenses; other expenses as determined.
Website: www.ictp.trieste.it/~twows/postgrad.html

Research in Training Award
Sponsor: Wilderness Medicine Society.
Target applicant: A medical resident, fellow, or PhD student.
Location: Not specified.
Description: Award recipients will conduct well-defined projects likely to result in a substantive contribution to the field of wilderness and environmental medicine.
Stipend: Up to $5,000.
Website: www.wms.org

Sara's Wish Scholarship Fund
Sponsor: Sara's Wish Foundation.
Target applicant: An extraordinary young woman who is committed to making the world a better place by fully participating in it.
Location: All areas of the world.
Description: Sara Christie Schewe was killed while in her junior year at college in a bus crash in India while participating in the Semester at Sea Program. Sara's Wish Foundation educational travel scholarships are awarded to young women who perpetuate Sara's ideals.
Stipend: TBD. Previous awardees have received between $1,000 and $1,500.
Website: www.saraswish.org

Service Learning Program (SLP) in China
Sponsor: Wang Foundation.
Target applicant: A U.S. student in any major and at any level of under-graduate or graduate study.
Location: China.
Description: The primary task of SLP participants is teaching conversational English to local teachers and public officials in 22 of China's provinces. At the same time, the program helps U.S. participants learn first-hand about the real China by delivering community services on a personal level. U.S. students also have the opportunity to conduct research in areas of their academic interest. The SLP includes 1 week of orientation in Beijing, followed by 4 weeks residing and working in the assigned site.
Stipend: In-country costs are offset by Wang Foundation scholarships awarded to all participants admitted into the program. The scholarship covers room and board expenses incurred inside China, including the week of orientation in Beijing and the 4 weeks at the service site, plus public ground transportation to and from the service site.
Website: wangfoundation.net/service_learning.htm

Shine-a-light Fellowship
Sponsor: Shine-a-light.
Target applicant: A graduate student in medicine, psychology, or other field who can help agencies working with street kids.
Location: Latin America.
Description: Three-month fellowship to work with street children.
Stipend: $1,500 for airfare and housing.
Website: www.shinealight.org

Undergraduate Students

AWC Scholarship
Sponsor: American Women's Club in Stockholm (AWC).
Target applicant: American female citizen, 18 years or older, currently living in the United States.
Location: Sweden.
Description: The AWC makes it possible for American women to study in Sweden. The scholarship is awarded for academic excellence. The applicant must be accepted for a period of study or research at a Swedish educational institute. All academic fields are eligible.
Stipend: $1,500 travel grant.
Website: www.awcstockholm.org

Global Health Council Internship Program
Sponsor: Global Health Council.
Target applicant: A graduate or undergraduate student at an accredited university.
Location: Washington, DC, or White River Junction, Vermont.
Description: The GHC internships offer students unique learning experiences in advocating and supporting programs that improve health around the world; 30 hours per week over 12 weeks.
Stipend: $200 per month.
Website: www.globalhealth.org

Global Health Fellows
Sponsor: U.S. Agency for International Development (USAID).
Target applicant: An outstanding student or mid-career changer interested in pursuing a career in international development.
Location: Washington, DC.
Description: Ten-week summer internships at USAID's Bureau for Global Health in various areas.

Stipend: Hourly rate based on education and experience
Website: www.ghfp.net

HIVCorps
Sponsor: Centre for Infectious Diseases Research in Zambia (CIDRZ).
Target applicant: A pre-medical or pre-M.P.H. student (including one graduating from a post-baccalaureate program), a medical or nursing student, or a recent M.P.H. graduate who wishes to gain international experience.
Location: Zambia.
Description: This 10- to 12-month program is designed to provide students and recent graduates with the opportunity to participate in international HIV programs and research initiatives.
Stipend: Monthly stipend of $1,000 to cover basic living expenses and airfare to Zambia. Housing, costs related to program activities, and local and emergency evacuation insurance is also provided.
Website: www.hopkinsglobalhealth.org/resources/funding/HIVCorps.pdf

IES Scholarships and Aid
Sponsor: Institute for International Education of Students (IES).
Target applicant: A student enrolled at any one of the approximately 160 leading public and private U.S. colleges and universities.
Location: IES offers nearly 30 programs in 16 countries.
Description: The IES mission is to provide students and U.S. colleges and universities with high-quality academic study abroad programs that foster intercultural development. Various programs feature courses in health and medicine. Summer, semester, and academic year options are available.
Stipend: IES offers scholarships and need-based financial aid up to $3,000 for semester and full-year programs and up to $1,000 for summer programs.
Website: www.iesabroad.org

Mabelle Arole Fellowship
Sponsor: JSI Research and Training Institute, Inc.
Target applicant: A U.S. citizen or permanent resident who has been accepted to medical school, but has not yet begun.
Location: Jamkhed, India.
Description: One-year program at the Comprehensive Rural Health

Project in Jamkhed, India, working with a primary health care project.
Stipend: Quarterly stipend covers housing, living expenses, and round-trip airfare.
Website: www.amsa.org

NSEP David L. Boren Undergraduate Scholarships
Sponsor: National Security Education Programs (NSEP).
Target applicant: A U.S. citizen who is enrolled in a post-secondary institution accredited by the U.S. Department of Education.
Location: See website for preferred countries.
Description: The NSEP awards focus on geographical areas, languages, and fields of study deemed critical to U.S. national security. The scope of national security includes: sustainable development, environmental degradation, global disease and hunger, population growth and migration, and economic competitiveness. A foreign language component is required for all study abroad proposals. The scholarships include a NSEP service requirement. Full academic year proposals are given preference.
Stipend: Up to $20,000 for a full academic year, $10,000 for a semester, $8,000 for a summer.
Website: www.iie.org/programs/nsep

NYU in London Science Scholarship
Sponsor: New York University (NYU).
Target applicant: A student from an institution other than NYU who is pursuing a major or minor in premed or a science-related field.
Location: London, England.
Description: The academic program at NYU in London has been designed to give undergraduates majoring in the sciences and pre-health professions options that may enable them to continue their curriculum without interruption while studying abroad. The curriculum is a series of courses designed to replicate the requirements of the NYU home departments.
Stipend: A $2,000 scholarship (in the form of tuition credit) is awarded on the basis of merit and is available to students from other institutions. Students whose home school has an institutional relationship with NYU are not eligible to apply.
Website: www.nyu.edu

Paul W. Zuccaire Internship Program
Sponsor: Pasteur Foundation.
Target applicant: An applicant must (1) be an undergraduate with a strong interest in biosciences and biomedical research; (2) have completed 2 full years of college course work by the time the internship commences; and (3) not yet have received an undergraduate degree at the time of application. Open to U.S. citizens only.
Location: Paris, France.
Description: The goal of the internship is to encourage students in the pursuit of a scientific career and to expose them to an international laboratory experience. Internships are for 10 weeks.
Stipend: $4,000 living allowance and $300 subsidy to defray cost of travel and insurance.
Website: www.pasteurfoundation.org

Sara's Wish Scholarship Fund
Sponsor: Sara's Wish Foundation.
Target applicant: An extraordinary young woman committed to making the world a better place by fully participating in it.
Location: All areas of the world.
Description: Sara Christie Schewe was killed while in her junior year at college in a bus crash in India while participating in the Semester at Sea Program. Sara's Wish Foundation educational travel scholarships are awarded to young women who perpetuate Sara's ideals.
Stipend: TBD. Previous awardees have received $1,000 to $1,500.
Website: www.saraswish.org

Service Learning Program (SLP) in China
Sponsor: Wang Foundation.
Target applicant: A U.S. student in any major and at any level of undergraduate or graduate study.
Location: China.
Description: The primary task of SLP participants is teaching conversational English to local teachers and public officials in 22 of China's provinces. At the same time, the program helps U.S. participants learn first-hand about the real China by delivering community services on a personal level. U.S. students also have the opportunity to conduct research in areas of their academic interest. The SLP includes 1 week of orientation in Beijing, followed by 4 weeks residing and working in the assigned site.

Stipend: In-country costs are offset by Wang Foundation scholarships awarded to all participants admitted into the program. The scholarship covers room and board expenses incurred inside China, including the week of orientation in Beijing and the 4 weeks at the service site, plus public ground transportation to and from the service site.
Website: wangfoundation.net

Thomas J. Watson Fellowship
Sponsor: Thomas J. Watson Foundation.
Target applicant: A graduating senior at one of the participating institutions.
Location: A foreign country where the recipient has not lived or studied for a significant length of time.
Description: The Watson Fellowship is a 1-year grant for independent study and travel outside the United States. It is awarded to graduating seniors nominated by the participating institutions. Nominees must submit a proposal for a project that is creative, feasible, and personally significant.
Stipend: $25,000 ($35,000 for fellows accompanied by a spouse or dependent child) for the fellowship year. The foundation will reimburse the equivalent of 12 months of payments on outstanding institutional and federally guaranteed (Perkins, Stafford) loans. The fellow is responsible for making the payments.
Website: www.watsonfellowship.org

Scholars and Professionals (Doctorate Level)

AAAS Science and Technology Policy Fellowship
Sponsor: American Association for the Advancement of Science.
Target applicant: A holder of a PhD, MD, or equivalent doctoral-level degree in science, engineering, or relevant interdisciplinary field.
Location: U.S. government agency.
Description: This is an internationally oriented public policy learning experience to make practical contributions to effective use of scientific and technical knowledge in foreign affairs and international development programs of the U.S. government.
Stipend: Based on education and training; estimated $67,000 to $87,000 annually.
Website: fellowships.aaas.org

Advanced Study or Research in Scandinavia
Sponsor: American-Scandinavian Foundation.
Target applicant: A U.S. citizen or permanent resident who has completed undergraduate education.
Location: Denmark, Finland, Iceland, Norway, or Sweden.
Description: Applicants must have a well-defined research or study project that makes a stay in Scandinavia essential. Awards are made in all fields.
Stipend: Awards support project-related costs, including maintenance and travel. Fellowship awards (for year-long study) are up to $20,000 and grants (for 1 to 3 months of study) are normally $4,000.
Website: www.amscan.org

ASPH/CDC Allan Rosenfield Global Health Fellowship Program
Sponsor: Association of Schools of Public Health (ASPH), with support from the Centers for Disease Control (CDC).
Target applicant: A recent graduate of an ASPH member accredited school of public health or early career professional with a graduate degree from an ASPH member school of public health.
Location: CDC headquarters in Atlanta, Georgia, as well as various international locations.
Description: The purpose of the fellowship is to enhance the training of graduates of the schools of public health with an interest in global health to experience and participate in aspects of global surveillance, monitoring and evaluation, epidemiology, strategic information, program management, and HIV prevention, and to accelerate their careers as leaders in global public health. The duration of the fellowship is 1 to 2 years.
Stipend: $35,370.
Website: www.asph.org

Burroughs Wellcome Fund/ASTMH Post-doctoral Fellowship in Tropical Infectious Disease
Sponsor: American Society of Tropical Medicine and Hygiene (ASTMH).
Target applicant: A North American clinician-scientist enrolled in (or accepted by) an accredited fellowship program.
Location: United States or Canada and a tropical/developing area.
Description: The purpose of the BWF/ASTMH fellowship is to stimu-

late or sustain research in tropical infectious diseases. Funding is available for two 12-month periods. At least 3 months of each year are spent working in a tropical or developing area.
Stipend: $65,000 per year for 2 years to cover stipend, fringe benefits, and health insurance. In the second year, $10,000 is also available for supplies, communications, and travel expenses.
Website: www.astmh.org

Christine Mirzayan Science and Technology Policy Graduate Fellowship Program
Sponsor: National Academies.
Target applicant: A current graduate student or postdoc or scholar who has completed graduate studies or post-doctoral research within the past 5 years in any of the following fields: a physical, biological, or social science or any field of engineering, medicine or health, or veterinary medicine, as well as business, law, education, or other professional programs.
Location: Washington, DC.
Description: The program is designed to engage graduate science, engineering, medical, veterinary, business, and law students in the analysis that informs the creation of science and technology, and government.
Stipend: $5,300 for the 10-week program.
Website: www7.nationalacademies.org

Embassy of Belgium Study and Research Fellowships
Sponsor: Embassy of Belgium.
Target applicant: A U.S. citizen with a bachelor's or master's degree, not older than 35 years, and without other Belgian sources of income.
Location: Flanders, Belgium.
Description: Fellowships are granted for study or research at institutions recognized by the Flemish community in various fields, including medicine. Fellowship duration is 10 months.
Stipend: Monthly stipend of approximately 720 Euros, reimbursement of the tuition fee, and health and liability insurance.
Website: www.diplobel.us

Fulbright Program for U.S. Scholars
Sponsor: U.S. Department of State.
Target applicant: A U.S. scholar or professional in any discipline.

Location: Many available countries.
Description: A variety of grants are awarded for periods of 2 weeks to a full academic year for specified activities (approximately 1,600 awards per year).
Stipend: Grants include airfare, related expenses, and an honorarium. Host institutions may cover in-country costs for lodging, meals, and transportation.
Website: www.cies.org/Fulbright_programs.htm

Guest Scholarship Programme
Sponsor: Swenka Institutet (Swedish Institute).
Target applicant: An individual in advanced-level studies in any subject.
Location: Sweden.
Description: The scholarships are intended to finance advanced university-level courses or the middle or concluding portion of the studies required for a PhD degree, with the studies begun outside of Sweden, or post-doctoral research or studies for holders of a PhD degree.
Stipend: Unspecified.
Website: www.si.se

Guggenheim Foundation Research Grants
Sponsor: Harry Frank Guggenheim Foundation.
Target applicant: A researcher in the natural or social sciences or the humanities who is studying the causes, manifestations, and control of violence, aggression, and dominance.
Location: Not specified.
Description: The foundation awards research grants to individuals for individual projects. Requests will be considered for research for 1 to 3 years and may include field work.
Stipend: $15,000 to 30,000 for 1 to 2 years.
Website: www.hfg.org

HFSC Long-Term Fellowship
Sponsor: Human Frontier Science Program.
Target applicant: A PhD researcher early in a career in the life sciences.
Location: Many countries.
Description: This fellowship is for basic research and training in a new area of research in an outstanding laboratory in another country.

Stipend: Living allowance, research and travel allowance, plus other allowances.
Website: www.hfsp.org

HFSP Short-Term Fellowship
Sponsor: Human Frontier Science Program.
Target applicant: A basic science researcher early in a career who wishes to work for a short period in a laboratory in another country.
Location: Many countries.
Description: The fellowship funds basic research focused on elucidating the complex mechanisms of living organisms; emphasis is placed on approaches that involve scientific exchanges across national boundaries.
Stipend: Travel and living expenses.
Website: www.hfsp.org

IFUW International Awards
Sponsor: International Federation of University Women (IFUW).
Target applicant: A woman graduate who is a member of one of IFUW's national federations and associations or an IFUW international member.
Location: Any country other than the one in which the applicant was educated or habitually resides.
Description: Fellowships, 8 to 12 months long, are offered for the second and subsequent years of a doctoral program and for post-doctoral studies. Grants are for a minimum of 2 months of work.
Stipend: Based on the award.
Website: www.ifuw.org

India Elective Travel Scholarship
Sponsor: American Association of Physicians of Indian Origin (AAPI).
Target applicant: A student, resident, or fellow in an accredited U.S. scholar training program; must be a member of the AAPI medical student, resident, and fellows section.
Location: India.
Description: Three scholarships are awarded to subsidize educational electives in India.
Stipend: $1,000.
Website: www.aapimsr.org

International Research Scientist Development Award (IRSDA)
Sponsor: U.S. Department of Health and Human Services.
Target applicant: A U.S. citizen, non-citizen national, or individual lawfully admitted for U.S. permanent residence who has earned a doctoral, dental, or medical degree within 7 years of the application receipt date.
Location: Developing countries.
Description: The award supports the recipient for a 3- to 4-year period of collaboration with a U.S. mentor and an established developing country mentor with the purpose to build research capacity to address global health research priorities.
Stipend: Total award is expected to be $250,000 to $500,000.
Website: grants.nih.gov

Johnson Short Term Medical Missions Fund
Sponsor: Christian Medical and Dental Associations (CMDA).
Target applicant: A resident or fellow; must be a CMDA member.
Location: Developing countries.
Description: The purpose of the fund is to encourage participation in a missionary medical or dental preceptorship.
Stipend: Up to $1,000 per person or $2,000 per married couple.
Website: www.cmdahome.org

JSPS Fellowships
Sponsor: Japan Society for the Promotion of Science (JSPS).
Target applicant: A PhD student or researcher who is a United Kingdom national and is studying or has graduated from a U.K. institution or is currently conducting research at that institution.
Location: Japan.
Description: The program allows applicants to conduct research with Japanese colleagues in a designated area. A variety of short- and long-term fellowships are available.
Stipend: Airfare, maintenance allowance, and domestic research travel allowance, with additional support provided for longer-term positions.
Website: www.jsps.org

Lindbergh Grants
Sponsor: Charles A. and Anne Morrow Lindbergh Foundation.
Target applicant: A U.S. citizen who is conducting research or educational projects in any of various categories, including health.

Location: Many available locations.
Description: Grants are provided to men and women whose individual initiative and work in a wide spectrum of disciplines furthers the Lindberghs' vision of a balance between the advance of technology and the preservation of the natural and human environment.
Stipend: Up to $10,580 (a symbolic amount representing the cost of the *Spirit of St Louis*).
Website: www.lindberghfoundation.org

NEW AID Scholarship
Sponsor: NEW AID Foundation.
Target applicant: A public health graduate student or a scientist early in her or his career.
Location: Latin America, Asia, Africa, or Eastern Europe. Other areas evaluated on a case-by-case basis.
Description: Stipends are awarded to conduct public health research abroad on the abandoned infectious diseases of marginalized populations.
Stipend: Up to $4,500 for individual stipends; approximately $8,000 plus airfare for research grants.
Website: www.newaid.org

Pasteur Foundation Post-Doctoral Fellowship Program
Sponsor: Pasteur Foundation.
Target applicant: A post-doctoral researcher who is a U.S. citizen and not currently living in France.
Location: Paris, France.
Description: The Pasteur Foundation brings U.S. researchers to work in Institut Pasteur laboratories in Paris. The institute's administration seeks to develop international scientific exchanges to ensure the vitality and quality of Institut Pasteur labs. Candidates are expected to commit to a 3-year stay.
Stipend: $45,000 stipend plus $15,000 bench fees to support the research per year for a term of 3 years.
Website: www.pasteurfoundation.org

Robert E. Shope International Fellowship
Sponsor: American Society of Tropical Medicine and Hygiene.
Target applicant: A full-time post-doctoral fellow with a position at a North American institution who studies tropical infectious disease in arbovirology and/or emerging tropical infectious diseases.

Location: Open.
Description: The work is to be in a laboratory in the tropics to pursue studies in arbovirology and/or emerging tropical infectious diseases.
Stipend: $10,000 to help defray travel costs, living expenses, and/or research abroad.
Website: www.astmh.org

SDE/GWIS Fellowships
Sponsor: Sigma Delta Epsilon (SDE) and Graduate Women in Science (GWIS).
Target applicant: An SDE/GWIS member who is enrolled as a graduate student or engaged in post-doctoral or early-stage junior faculty academic research who has demonstrated financial need.
Location: Unspecified.
Description: The SDE/GWIS Fellowships are academic year awards that can be used for applied or basic research. The overall purpose is to increase the fundamental knowledge of the sciences, and increase the visibility of women with careers in scientific research.
Stipend: Based on the award category, up to $4,000.
Website: www.gwis.org

Yale/Johnson and Johnson Physician Scholars in International Health Program
Sponsor: Yale University and Johnson and Johnson.
Target applicant: A medical resident or career physician.
Location: Developing countries.
Description: Physicians-in-training and career physicians will spend 4- to 8-week rotations in overseas sites. Rotations are directed at clinical experiences, service, and teaching, as opposed to research.
Stipend: $1,000 to $5,000 travel award received on completion of the rotation.
Website: www.medicine.yale.edu

Scholars and Professionals (Non-Doctorate Level)

AAUW International Fellowships
Sponsor: American Association of University Women.
Target applicant: A woman who is a U.S. citizen or permanent resident for graduate or post-graduate study.
Location: Any country, other than the recipient's own.
Description: Fellowships are awarded for full-time study or research. Home

Country Project Grants support community-based projects designed to improve the lives of women and girls in the fellow's home country.
Stipend: $18,000 to $30,000 for fellowships, $5,000 to $7,000 for Home Country Project Grants.
Website: www.aauw.org

AIF Service Corps Fellowship
Sponsor: American India Foundation (AIF).
Target applicant: A U.S. citizen or permanent resident, aged between 21 and 35, with an undergraduate degree and strong interest in India's development sector.
Location: India.
Description: This is a 10-month fellowship working with a non-govern-mental organization in India in the areas of education, livelihood, and public health.
Stipend: Monthly stipend, housing allowance, food and transport allowance, travel to and from India, language training allowance; mis-cellaneous costs.
Website: www.aifoundation.org

ASPH/CDC Allan Rosenfield Global Health Fellowship Program
Sponsor: Association of Schools of Public Health (ASPH), with support from the Centers for Disease Control (CDC).
Target applicant: A recent graduate of an ASPH member accredited school of public health or an early career professional with a graduate degree from an ASPH member school of public health.
Location: CDC headquarters in Atlanta, Georgia, as well as various international locations.
Description: The purpose of the fellowship is to enhance the training of graduates of the schools of public health with an interest in global health to experience and participate in aspects of global surveillance, monitor-ing and evaluation, epidemiology, strategic information, program man-agement, and HIV prevention, and to accelerate their careers as leaders in global public health. The duration of the fellowship is 1 to 2 years.
Stipend: $35,370.
Website: www.asph.org

Fulbright Program for U.S. Scholars
Sponsor: U.S. Department of State.
Target applicant: A U.S. scholar or professional in any discipline.

Location: Many available countries.

Description: A variety of grants are awarded for periods of 2 weeks to a full academic year for specified activities (approximately 1,600 awards per year).

Stipend: Grants include airfare, related expenses, and an honorarium. Host institutions may cover in-country costs for lodging, meals, and transportation.

Website: www.cies.org/Fulbright_programs.htm

Global Health Fellows

Sponsor: US Agency for International Development (USAID).

Target applicant: An outstanding student or mid-career changer interested in pursuing a career in international development.

Location: Washington, DC.

Description: Ten-week summer internships located at USAID's Bureau for Global Health in various areas.

Stipend: Hourly rate based on education and experience.

Website: www.ghfp.net

Indicorps Service Fellowship

Sponsor: Indicorps.

Target applicant: A professional of Indian origin who has a university degree or 5 years of equivalent work experience.

Location: India.

Description: This is a public service program for projects that address particular development challenges and are created and defined in partnership with local developmental experts.

Stipend: Room, board, and fellowship-related travel are provided.

Website: www.indicorps.org

International Development Fellows Program (IDFP)

Sponsor: Catholic Relief Services (CRS).

Target applicant: An individual interested in a career in international relief and development. Must have relevant work experience and professional proficiency in French, Spanish, or Portuguese. A master's degree in a relevant field preferred.

Location: CRS operates in 99 countries around the world.

Description: The goal of the IDFP is to place fellows in positions where they can draw on their previous education and work experience, while broadening their skills. Assignments are for 1 year.

Stipend: Monthly stipend based on location, cost of living adjustment, housing, airfare, vacation, insurance.
Website: www.crs.org

International Health Youth Internships Program
Sponsor: Canadian Society for International Health.
Target applicant: A citizen or permanent resident of Canada, between 19 and 30 years of age.
Location: To be determined.
Description: The program offers volunteer placement in developing countries to young adults with appropriate skills in information and communication technologies for 6-week periods. Placements are with health organizations and health and development agencies.
Stipend: To be determined.
Website: www.csih.org

International Fellows Program
Sponsor: Center on Philanthropy and Civil Society.
Target applicant: A young scholar-practitioner in the non-profit sector interested in building third-sector capacity in the United States and overseas.
Location: New York City.
Description: Leadership training through applied research and professional mentorships.
Stipend: Cost of tuition, accommodations, travel, and $1,300 per month.
Website: philanthropy.org

Luce Scholars Program
Sponsor: Henry Luce Foundation.
Target applicant: The candidate must be a U.S. citizen who has received at least a bachelor's degree and is no more than 29 years old. Those who have significant experience in Asia or Asian studies are not eligible for the program. Nominees must have a record of high achievement, outstanding leadership ability, and a clearly defined career interest with evidence of potential for professional accomplishment.
Location: Asia.
Description: The Luce Scholars Program provides stipends and internships for 18 Americans to live and work in Asia each year. Placement and support services are provided by the Asia Foundation. Sixty-seven

U.S. colleges and universities are eligible to make nominations for the program.
Stipend: Basic stipend plus cost-of-living allowance and basic housing allowance where necessary.
Website: www.hluce.org

Roma Initiatives Fellowship
Sponsor: Open Society Institute (OSI) and Soros Foundations Network.
Target applicant: An individual with a university degree active in the field of Roma rights.
Location: Available in Bulgaria, Croatia, the Czech Republic, Hungary, Macedonia, Romania, Serbia and Montenegro, and Slovakia.
Description: Individuals work with an OSI mentor to develop a range of initiatives regarding a variety of topics, including health policy, that are important for the inclusion of Roma in society. Fellowships are generally for a 12-month period.
Stipend: According to the agreed initiative.
Website: www.soros.org

Residents and Fellows

AMWA Overseas Assistance Grant
Sponsor: American Medical Women's Association (AMWA)/American Women's Hospitals Service.
Target applicant: A national AMWA student or resident member. Medical students must be completing their second, third, or fourth year at an accredited U.S. medical school.
Location: Off-campus setting where the medically neglected will benefit.
Description: Six weeks to 1 year will be spent in a sponsored program, which will serve the needs of the medically underserved.
Stipend: Up to $1,500.
Website: www.amwa-doc.org

Don and Elizabeth Hillman International Health Grant
Sponsor: Canadian Paediatric Society (CPS).
Target applicant: A resident or fellow in a Canadian pediatric postgraduate training program and member of the CPS International Health Section.
Location: Unspecified.

Description: The grant supports a clinical or research elective of at least 4 weeks in length that relates to child health.
Stipend: $750.
Website: www.cps.ca

India Elective Travel Scholarship
Sponsor: American Association of Physicians of Indian Origin (AAPI).
Target applicant: A student, resident, or fellow in an accredited U.S. scholar training program; must be a member of the AAPI medical student, resident, and fellows section.
Location: India.
Description: The scholarship provides three scholarships to subsidize educational electives in India.
Stipend: $1,000.
Website: www.aapimsr.org

International Travel Grants
Sponsor: American Academy of Pediatrics.
Target applicant: A pediatric resident.
Location: Developing world.
Description: The grants are awarded to categorical pediatric or combined-training pediatric residents who wish to complete a clinical pediatric elective in the developing world.
Stipend: $500 grant.
Website: www.aap.org

Johnson Short Term Medical Missions Fund
Sponsor: Christian Medical and Dental Associations (CMDA).
Target applicant: A resident or fellow; must be a CMDA member.
Location: Developing countries.
Description: The purpose of the fund is to encourage participation in a missionary medical or dental preceptorship.
Stipend: Up to $1,000 per person or $2,000 per married couple.
Website: www.cmdahome.org

MAP International Medical Fellowship
Sponsor: MAP International.
Target applicant: A third- or fourth-year medical student, resident, or intern.

Location: Mission agency or hospital that has an outreach among the poor in a rural or urban setting.
Description: MAP provides exposure in a Christian context to the health, social, and cultural characteristics of a developing community. Students must spend at least 8 weeks in the field; 6 weeks for residents and interns.
Stipend: Round-trip airfare to destination.
Website: www.map.org

Research in Training Award
Sponsor: Wilderness Medicine Society.
Target applicant: A medical resident, fellow, or PhD graduate student.
Location: Not specified.
Description: Award recipients will conduct well-defined projects likely to result in a substantive contribution to the field of wilderness and environmental medicine.
Stipend: Up to $5,000.
Website: www.wms.org

Yale/Johnson and Johnson Physician Scholars in International Health Program
Sponsor: Yale University and Johnson and Johnson.
Target applicant: A medical resident or career physician.
Location: Developing countries.
Description: Physicians-in-training and career physicians will spend 4- to 8-week rotations in overseas sites. Rotations are directed at clinical experiences, service, and teaching, as opposed to research.
Stipend: $1,000 to $5,000 travel award received on completion of the rotation.
Website: www.medicine.yale.edu

Loan Repayment Programs

Dr and Mrs Ernest Steury Medical Student Scholarship Fund
Sponsor: Christian Medical and Dental Associations.
Target applicant: A U.S. citizen in the first or second year of training in an American institution, working toward an MD or DO degree, with desire to serve in medical missions.
Location: Foreign or domestic mission site.
Description: The fund provides assistance with the tuition of medical

students who are committed to a career in foreign or domestic medical missions.
Stipend: $25,000 per year, renewed on a yearly basis until graduation from a medical or osteopathy school.
Website: www.cmdahome.org

Project MedSend Student Loan Repayment Grant
Sponsor: MedSend.
Target applicant: An upper-level health care student committed to serve as a medical missionary.
Location: Medically underserved areas of the world.
Description: Project MedSend offers grants to repay student loans owed by health care professionals while serving as medical missionaries.
Stipend: Based on monthly student loan payments.
Website: www.medsend.org

Other Opportunities

CFHI International Fellows Program
Sponsor: Child Family Health International (CFHI).
Target applicant: A past participant of a CFHI international program.
Location: Many international locations.
Description: Fellows work with local coordinators to prepare host communities for the arrival of CFHI students and to plan the 4-week clinical rotations for a period of 10 weeks.
Stipend: Round-trip airfare to host country from San Francisco, daily stipend of $20, general stipend of $300 paid on completion of reporting formalities at the end of the 10-week fellowship.
Website: www.cfhi.org

Change Ambassadors Grant
Sponsor: Travelocity.
Target applicant: Anyone interested in volunteer travel (minimum age 18).
Location: Worldwide sites offered by Travelocity's designated volunteer travel partners.
Description: Travelocity's Travel for Good program awards grants to subsidize volunteer vacations. Special consideration is given to those who have demonstrated long-term contributions through volunteering, and to those who do not have the financial means to take a volunteer vacation on their own.

Stipend: Up to $5,000 for transportation.
Website: leisure.travelocity.com/Promotions/0,,TRAVELOCITY%
7C3915%7Cvacations_main,00.html

Christiansen Grant
Sponsor: InterExchange Foundation.
Target applicant: An individual who has sought out and arranged her or
his own work abroad program, with preference to those with limited
international travel experience and longer programs.
Location: Not specified.
Description: The proposed program must emphasize a work component
and cannot be independent research projects. Recipients will be
selected based on intent.
Stipend: $10,000 for 12+ months; $5,000 for 6+ months; $2,500 for 6+
weeks.
Website: www.interexchange.org

GHM Short-term Mission Volunteers
Sponsor: Global Health Ministries (GHM).
Target applicant: A volunteer for short-term mission service in overseas
Lutheran health care facilities.
Location: Overseas Lutheran health care partners.
Description: Volunteers work with short-term training, service, and pro-
gram development projects.
Stipend: Partial subsidies for expenses.
Website: www.ghm.org

ProWorld Scholarships
Sponsor: ProWorld.
Target applicant: A participant in ProWorld's summer and fall programs.
Location: Varies.
Description: Scholarships are based on need and merit and are available
for all of ProWorld's summer and fall programs offered in various
areas, including health care.
Stipend: $1,000 and $2,000.
Website: www.myproworld.org/costs/scholarships.htm

Reebok Human Rights Award
Sponsor: Reebok Human Rights Foundation.
Target applicant: An individual 30 years of age or younger who is work-

ing on an issue that directly relates to the U.N. Universal Declaration of Human Rights.
Location: Unspecified.
Description: The Reebok Human Rights Award helps activists achieve their goals by bringing international attention to the injustices that they have been fighting. Women and men of all races, ethnic groups, nationalities, and religious backgrounds are eligible.
Stipend: $50,000 grant to further the work of each award recipient.
Website: www.reebok.com

Travelers' Diarrhea Vaccine Study
Sponsor: Iomai Corporation.
Target applicant: A healthy male or female, aged 18–64.
Location: Mexico or Guatemala.
Description: The Iomai Corporation is conducting a Phase 2 trial of a travellers' diarrhea vaccine. Participants in the field study must be travelling to sites in and around Cuernavaca or Guadalajara, Mexico, or Antigua, Guatemala.
Stipend: Up to $900.
Website: www.trekstudy.com

8 Trip Planning and Preparations

One of the most important aspects in achieving an excellent global health experience is proper trip planning and preparation. There are many considerations to take into account before embarking on an international experience. A well-planned trip can avoid a great deal of hardship or disappointment later. It is especially important to consider that it often takes much longer than you expect to prepare for a trip, including delays in getting visas and work permits, difficulties in registering for medical practice, and difficulties in communicating with host countries (although e-mail and Internet access has made this significantly easier). The following topics are covered in detail throughout this chapter:

- Orientation
- Duties and Responsibilities
- Language
- Travel Visa and Work Permit
- Travel Plans
- Personal Health
- Personal Safety
- Health Insurance and Baggage Insurance
- Accommodations and Food
- Medical Licence and Registration
- Cost
- Equipment and Supplies
- Communications
- Post-trip Debriefing

Orientation

Proper orientation is often an aspect of trip planning and preparation that is neglected. It is insufficient to just buy an airplane ticket and show up in a country. Certain aspects of culture and language, such as simple greetings or avoiding touching a monk's robes in a Buddhist country, should be learned. This could minimize violating cultural taboos and help increase, or at least not hinder, acceptance into a culture and society. Part of the orientation should focus on what you expect to learn and achieve while abroad to clarify your expectations and to look at alternatives if plans don't go as you had in mind. You should look at possible assistance that you require such as translation services, drivers to locations, etc. And perhaps the most important aspect you should do is ask yourself this simple question: What would be useful to leave behind that will help my hosts? Even the most experienced practitioners should take the time to orient, especially if travelling to a new location for the first time.

Before departing, it is important to learn as much as possible about the host country and its culture, and the host organization and its global health work or projects. Some universities provide courses for overseas travel. One of the best ways to familiarize yourself is to contact the embassy of the country that you're going to; find a contact from that country who lives nearby to help orient you to your international destination. However, much can be achieved simply by learning about a country from the Internet, from a guidebook (such as the *Lonely Planet* series), or by asking people with knowledge about your country and locale (see Table 8.1).

Often, a recently returned volunteer or worker can provide the most up-to-date advice and a more honest description of the place and work. If possible, ask the organization or hospital for the contact information of a person who has recently returned from the site. You should inquire from the contacts about their experiences and listen to any suggestions they may be able to offer about the site and work.

However, there is nothing like first-hand experience, and most of your learning will occur on the ground. Get to know the key contacts in the country, and if possible, settle living arrangements and transportation for the duration of your stay.

Try to arrive in the host country a few days before the actual start date in order to have some time to settle into the new environment. It is often

Table 8.1
25 Questions to Orientate Yourself

1 How many prominent individuals, historical figures, and politicians can you name from your host country?

2 What are the official languages of your host country? What are the social and political implications of these languages?

3 What are the major religions in your country? Is there an official state religion? What are the official dates of observance and/or ceremonies? Do people participate in them regularly?

4 What things are 'taboo' in society?

5 What is the official position of the state on HIV/AIDS? Does the community stigmatize people with HIV/AIDS?

6 What is the official position of the state on adultery? Polygamy? Homosexuality? Divorce?

7 What is the attitude towards drinking and smoking?

8 What are the major food types and dishes in this area?

9 If you're in the market, is the labelled price the final sale price or can you barter for a better price? If so, how is a sale concluded?

10 If you're invited for dinner, should you arrive early? On time? Or Late?

11 Do you need to bring gifts for dinner?

12 How do people greet one another? And how do they leave one another?

13 What leisure activities are there?

14 What is a normal work schedule?

15 How many children do people have on average? What games do children play?

16 How are children disciplined? Are they expected to be part of social events?

17 How are children recognized as turning into adults?

18 What kind of local transportation is available?

19 What is the history of the relationship between the host country and the United States or Canada?

20 Is military training compulsory? Male/Female? At what age and how long?

21 What health services are available? Where would the nearest location be?

22 What 'home treatments' are available for various diseases?

23 Is education free? Is education compulsory?

24 In schools, how important is learning by rote? Are there libraries? Books? Science labs? Sports equipment? Equal numbers of boys and girls? Do children drop out?

25 How does your wealth compare with that of the majority of people in this society?

useful in group situations to start off the in-country orientation with a fun event such as a safari or a local trip to get the group used to working with each other. Be sensitive to the gender and ethnic relationships of the health care workers and between the health care workers and community when learning about the culture and customs. Know when it is acceptable to treat or examine a patient of the opposite gender. If you are in doubt, then ask. These interactions are often different than in the United States or Canada, and it is better to ask than to start burning bridges.

Here are some questions to ask:

- What are my expectations? What do I expect to learn or achieve?
- What type of assistance do I require?
- Are there recently returned people that I could contact for information?
- What are possible living accommodations and transport from the airport once I arrive?
- Are there any resources to learn more about the local culture and beliefs?
- What can I expect to leave behind that would be useful or help my hosts?

Duties and Responsibilities

You should define your duties and responsibilities before leaving for a global health experience. If you are expecting to treat clinical patients, then you do not want to arrive at a host location and find that they expect you to simply transport patients around the hospital. You also want to take care not to overextend yourself or your abilities. Being put in a position for which you are not qualified is not good for you or the patients. Be prepared to tell your supervisor you are not comfortable and need more supervision when it is needed. The responsibilities and abilities of a fourth-year medical student from the United Kingdom are different from those of a fourth-year medical student from the United States. For clinicians, know how much call you have to take, what department you will be working in, and how much bedside and classroom teaching is expected. Duties and responsibilities are a balancing act of providing the necessary services to any host organization and your education. When on a humanitarian mission, where the needs seem to be endless, you may have to place a limit on how much work you will do. There will often be patients lined up for hundreds of metres to see you for medical care. Without imposing any limits, you could easily find yourself working 24 hours a day. Set your limits for your own health and well-being. You may need to remind yourself that you will not be able to help everyone.

Here are some questions to ask:

- What are my duties and responsibilities on this project or in the clinic?
- Will I be working with patients in a clinic? If so, in what capacity?

Language

Although many countries have English as their native language, language is a very important aspect to consider when seeking an international placement. Some clinical positions, such as surgery, may require less knowledge of the native language, or you may be able to function easily with the help of a hired translator. Oftentimes, there may be a local physician who has screened and scheduled surgical cases in advance of the trip, so all the visiting surgeon has to do is the surgery. However, most long-term placements require at least some basic knowledge of the native language. Some non-governmental organizations and humanitarian agencies will provide language training prior to departure or during the experience. It is always good to learn some basic phrases in the native language before you go.

In addition, if you have a family, you will need to take their education into consideration before choosing a placement. There are many good English-speaking foreign schools around the world, but you may want to take some material for additional home schooling. The best education for the children may be local schooling, where they can learn the culture and language, in combination with some material for home schooling.

Here are some questions to ask:

- What is the primary language or dialect used in the area?
- How proficient are the health care workers and patients with English?
- What resources are available to start learning the local language?
- Are there opportunities to receive language training in the host country?

Travel Visa and Work Permit

A valid passport is now required to travel anywhere in the world. A travel visa is required to visit many countries, particularly developing countries. Passport and visa information can be obtained from the U.S. State Department (www.state.gov) or the Canadian Department of Foreign Affairs and International Trade (www.dfait-maeci.gc.ca/index. aspx). The visa can then be obtained from the host country embassy or consulate office in the United States or Canada, and may be arranged with assistance from your host organization. The time and cost of obtaining a travel visa will vary, but the process can take up to 6 months, so planning ahead is imperative. Medical students will sometimes need an education visa, or student visa, rather than a tourist visa. An education visa can be expensive. For example, a student visa in South Africa costs approximately $250.

A work permit is usually required in addition to a visa for people who intend to be paid or reside in the host country for more than 3 months. Most governments regulate work permits to ensure that visitors are not taking employment from local host-country nationals. Most work permits are arranged within the host country, and may also be arranged with the assistance of your host organization. It is a good idea to make a copy of your passport and other important documents and carry them in a different piece of baggage in case you lose the originals.

It is also a good idea to bring passport photos, if you want to travel to other countries before or after your global health experience. Visas to other countries usually require up to four passport-sized photos.

Here are some questions to ask:

- Do I need a travel visa or work permit?
- How much time do I need to get a travel visa or work permit?
- Should I bring some additional small passport-sized photos?
- Have I made duplicate copies of key documents?
- Do I need to bring any other official documents?

Travel Plans

There are many travel agencies that can help arrange trips to anywhere in the world. Travel agents will be able to inform you how to travel cheaply, while also using the safest and most reliable travel routes. Your host may also be able to suggest the best route for safe and efficient travel. Although advice from travel agents is valuable, the cheapest tickets are commonly found on the Internet. In addition, purchasing tickets through agents outside the United States can often be less expensive. Nonetheless, it is helpful to compare several different travel agents and websites. If you are travelling with a group it is often best to use a travel agency that specializes in groups; this will ensure you will all travel together. You should share your travel plans with your hosts before departing, since it is often difficult to communicate with them immediately upon arrival in a country. The following is a list of online travel agents with low airfares and easy-to-use websites:

Air Travel Network
www.airtravel.net

Airfare.com
www.airfare.com

Airlines Consolidators
www.airlineconsolidator.com

AirTreks.com
www.airtreks.com

Booking Buddy
www.bookingbuddy.com

DiscountAirfares.com
www.etn.nl

Fly Cheap Abroad
www.flycheapabroad.com

Intra Tours
www.intratours.com

Latin Discount Air
www.latindiscountair.com

Mobissimo Travel
www.mobissimo.com

SideStep
www.sidestep.com

Sky Auction
www.skyauction.com

STA Travel
www.statravel.com

Student Universe
www.studentuniverse.com

Travel Price
www.travelprice.be

Travel Zoo
www.travelzoo.com

You may also want to consider doing some in-country orientation and tourism at the start of your visit. This can help you acclimatize to the area without the stress of being immediately thrust into your work or project. In addition, some advanced preparation for your travels will be very beneficial. It is always wise to have a good travel guidebook, such as the *Lonely Planet* or *Rough Guide*. These books can be found at most local bookstores or at online bookstores. You may also want to make plans to travel in the region after your global health experience. These plans are best made in advance to provide enough time to travel afterwards.

If time is not a pressing issue, an attractive alternative is to seek an open ticket, which allows you the flexibility to change the dates of return, as long as a seat is available.

Here are some questions to ask:

- Should I arrange my flights and travel or have a travel agent arrange the trip?
- Should I purchase an open ticket?
- What is the best route to take and where should I fly into?
- Are there particular holidays or election days I should avoid?
- Are there any particular guidebooks on the area that might be useful?

Personal Health

Visiting a travel medicine clinic before departure to obtain adequate vaccinations and malaria prophylactic medications, if needed, is important. Contact your local travel medicine clinic or colleagues at your hospital to arrange an appointment several months before departing. You should also learn which vaccinations and type of malaria prophylaxis will be best in your setting, as these recommendations can change regularly. The World Health Organization website (www.who.int/countries/en/) is an excellent source of information on disease and vaccination recommendations for each country. The U.S. Centers for Disease Control and Prevention have an excellent website (www. cdc.gov/travel) for the health of travellers and vaccination recommendations. In Canada, a list of travel clinics can be found at the Public Health Agency of Canada (www.phac-aspc.gc.ca/tmp-pmv/travel/clinic-eng.php). You should plan to start getting immunizations at least 4 months before departing, and become familiar with any side effects of the new medications you may need to take. The following list of organizations and websites can serve as a reference for travel medicine issues:

Travel Medicine
www.travmed.com

U.S. Centers for Disease Control and Prevention
www.cdc.gov

International Society of Travel Medicine
www.istm.org

The University of Wisconsin HealthLink
healthlink.mcw.edu/travel-medicine/

World Health Organization
www.who.int

Be sure to bring the medications you take on a regular basis, especially for any significant chronic conditions such as hypertension and diabetes. Make sure your personal medications are in their appropriate container to prevent any confusion. Plan to carry enough medication for your entire stay as well as some extra medication for any unanticipated travel delays. One unfortunate physician had brought just enough of his necessary steroid medication for his scheduled travel time. When political unrest delayed his departure from the host country, he ran out of his steroid medication and became very ill. Be sure this does not happen to you. Furthermore, your medications should be kept in your carry-on luggage, rather than placed in the checked luggage. Not having medications because of lost luggage is a common problem on cruise ships, and the medications are often difficult to replace with the limited pharmacy supply kept on-board. A list of your medications along with their dosages should be kept in a secure location. It is also important to consider bringing a first-aid kit, including bandages, tensors, personal clean needles, and gloves. Finally, it may be wise to travel with some prescription antibiotics such as ciprofloxacin, just in case you or someone in your family may need them in an emergency. This should also be discussed during your travel medicine clinic visit.

When you travel, find out the baggage allowance of the airline. If possible, fill the remainder of your luggage with medications for donation, and with equipment, books, and toys that can be given to your host-country nationals. Also take clothes in good condition that you no longer wear at home, and give them to the locals, clinics, or hospital.

Here are some questions to ask:

- What vaccinations do I need to receive?
- Will I be in a malaria-endemic region, and if so what prophylaxis is recommended?
- Should I take some antibiotics for treatment, in case I get sick?
- Do I have enough of my necessary medications for the trip and any unexpected delays?

Personal Safety

Personal safety is one of the most important, and often overlooked, aspects to consider during international travel. Pay attention to the recommendations of your hosts about safe places to travel, and perhaps more importantly, the unsafe locations to avoid. For the most part, local people will be very friendly and appreciative of you being there, but there are also people who want to take advantage of you and your money.

Prior to departing, or shortly after arriving in the host country, register with the U.S. embassy or the Canadian embassy. The U.S. State Department website (www.state.gov) maintains up-to-date information about safety in countries around the world, and you can now register the details of your travel on their web. The Canadian Department of Foreign Affairs and International Trade (www.voyage.gc.ca) has very good information for Canadian travellers. They will advise you of any political concerns, and know to look for you in case there is an evacuation or an emergency at home. You should also know how to contact them should you need their assistance. It may be helpful in many ways to organize a global health experience with a fellow student or co-worker, or work in a group. Together, you may be able to assist one another through tough situations.

Do common-sense things that you would do at home. The number one killer of volunteer overseas workers is motor vehicle accidents. While abroad, it is important to wear your seatbelt and take necessary precautions not to sit in open-air trucks. There are numerous reports of travellers dying abroad in motor vehicle accidents and getting thrown from the back of a pick-up truck during an accident. Be careful and wear your seatbelt!

Another important consideration while abroad is to be careful about sexually transmitted infections, including HIV/AIDS. Although there is a feeling of increased freedom while travelling abroad, precautions you would take at home should be used abroad. This includes abstinence as the best way to prevent HIV/AIDS. However, if you do participate in sexual activity, consider protecting methods including using a condom. Many overseas workers have contracted sexually transmitted infections while having unprotected sex while abroad.

If possible, try to obtain some local currency before your departure. If you cannot find local currency, local merchants often accept U.S. dollars. However, it is best to take many small bills because locals will often not want to make change or could take advantage of your lack of knowledge about the local currency. Also, you should bring some larger bills or traveller's checks for preferred exchange rates at banks. Credit cards are a wonderful alternative to bring for security purposes. Internationally recognized credit cards (Visa or MasterCard in many countries, and less frequently, American Express) allow for money to be transferred easily. Furthermore, credit cards are widely accepted in hotels, which allow for some money also to be transferred into local cash. Finally, ATM machines are now available in most countries, even developing countries, and are often the easiest method of obtaining local currency at the best exchange rate. Make sure your ATM card will work where you are going, and know where the locations are that accept your card before leaving.

Here are some questions to ask:

- Are there certain areas of the country or city that I should avoid?
- When and where should I register with the embassy?
- What is the contact information for the embassy or consulate in the host country?
- Do I have adequate protection if I engage in sexual activity?
- What is the best way to access my money while travelling or in the host country?

Health Insurance and Baggage Insurance

Most basic medical insurance does not cover treatment outside the United States or Canada. Most host organizations should be able to assist in obtaining health insurance and, if necessary, any medical treatment. It is highly recommended to have some medical insurance that would include medical evacuation insurance for any unexpected medical emergencies. There are many unexpected events that can occur, such as a motor vehicle accident, infectious disease, or a new medical disease that may occur at any time. If you become disabled or need surgery when abroad, then evacuation insurance will transport you to a suitable medical facility for the procedure. The cost is usually less than $75 per month and can be well worth the expense in the event of an unexpected medical crisis. The following is a list of personal health insurance programs for international work:

CSA Travel
www.csatravelprotection.com

International Student Insurance
www.internationalstudentinsurance.com

Medex Assist
www.medexassist.com

SOS International
www.sosinternational.com

Zain Jeewanjee Insurance Agency
www.jeewanjee.com

In Canada, the best places to look for travel insurance include bank and credit card companies, and the automobile associations, such as the Canadian Automobile Association (CAA).

Canadian Automobile Association
www.caa.ca

It is also important to consider acquiring baggage insurance to help refund money for lost equipment and clothing, and possibly provide money for delays in baggage arrival. Baggage insurance is usually expensive ($75) for the amount of money returned ($500–$1,000), so a consideration of the pluses and minuses should be taken into account.

Here are some questions to ask:

- Is medical insurance provided by the organization?
- What is the most common type of medical insurance used by the group?
- Where would I seek treatment in case of an emergency?
- Does my medical insurance include emergency evacuations?
- Do I require baggage insurance?

Accommodations and Food

More often than not, your host or host organization will assist in arranging appropriate accommodations. In many countries, this may be a house or an apartment. Sometimes this may consist of a dormitory setting, and you may be expected to share a room. Sometimes, you may be required to stay in a hotel or hostel, and you may have to bring your own mosquito net and/or sleeping bag. In some rural areas, you may need to sleep on the floor or bring your own cot. Know in advance where you will be sleeping, what sleeping materials you should bring, and what the cost may be. However, your host organization should be able to provide you with those details.

The host organization may also provide meals or at least discounted food in the cafeteria or at restaurants. There may also be a place to cook food where you will be staying. It can be difficult to eat every meal in a cafeteria or outside restaurants for a longer-term placement. The host organization will be able to direct you to where it is safe to buy food, and ask about which fruits and vegetables are safe to eat and which foods should be avoided.

If cooking on your own, it is important to boil water, and get fruits and vegetables that can be peeled and cooked to avoid contamination. You should also be aware about eating food from street vendors. There are many stories of travellers catching diarrhea on a long bus or car ride from contaminated food. Don't be one of those stories!

Here are some questions to ask:

- What accommodations are available?
- What is the approximate cost of accommodation and local food?

- Should I bring a mosquito net and/or sleeping bag?
- Is there a kitchen or room to cook meals?

Medical Licence and Registration

Having an approved medical licence is generally not required for medical students. Residents and allied medical personal may need to show a locally approved medical licence in order to see patients. The organization arranging your placement will often assist in determining when local medical licences are necessary and, if needed, help you obtain one. For short-term volunteer medical work, a host country typically does not require a local medical licence and may ask for a copy of your existing medical licence or proof of being a medical student. However, a problem may arise if the government medical council suspects you might want to stay and establish a private practice. In order to establish a private medical practice, you will typically be asked to provide a certified copy of your degree, current licence, a letter of good standing, and a letter from your host organization describing your plan and responsibility. This process usually takes a couple of months at a minimum and could last a year or longer. Whether you plan to provide short- or long-term medical care, it is valuable to bring all of these documents with you. Malpractice insurance is most often not a big issue elsewhere and is often covered by the host organization. Most medical schools will cover medical students when they are doing a rotation abroad. Finally, a Doctor of Osteopathic Medicine may not be recognized as a licensed medical physician in many countries, resulting in more obstacles in obtaining local medical licensure.

Here are some questions to ask:

- Do I need to obtain a local medical licence?
- If so, what paperwork should I bring with me?

Cost

The cost of any global health experience will vary considerably, and depend largely on the organization, length of stay, and cost of living. Many host organizations will accept volunteers for their projects, and thus the experience will mainly cost the price of your own travel and living expenses. Some organizations may also offer a free place to sleep. More academic centres may charge an administration fee, usually $100 to $500, to cover the cost of completing the necessary paperwork and documents. Other organizations may charge a fee to cover not only the administrative costs but to also help fund their projects.

Organizations that are in the business of setting up global health volunteer experiences may charge up to $5,000 per person for a 3- to 4-week project. These opportunities can be beneficial for people with limited time, because the organization will arrange nearly all of the travel and project logistics. Since these trips can be extremely beneficial to students with limited funds, additional student loans may be an option to help pay for this valuable global health opportunity.

To help fund some global health opportunities, please refer back to Chapter 7.

Here are some questions to ask:

- What are the costs involved with this trip and experience?
- Are there any scholarships or funding sources available?

Equipment and Supplies

When it comes to equipment, supplies, and personal effects, the first dictum is: Don't bring anything that you can't afford to lose!

Any medical provider should be prepared to bring personal basic medical equipment, such as a stethoscope, blood pressure cuff, ophthalmoscope/otoscope, scrubs, etc. However, the host organization may be able to supply some medical equipment, and it should be able to offer some guidance on equipment and supplies. Pens and paper are also at a premium and are always good to have on hand and can be left behind. In addition, toys for children are always well received, and can often help break down the cultural or language barriers.

A number of years ago, drug companies and organizations were dumping expired medications into developing countries. As a result, the World Health Organizations has adopted a policy on drug donation, called 'Guidelines for Drug Donation' (whqlibdoc.who.int/hq/1999/WHO_EDM_PAR_99.4.pdf). In brief, the policy states that one should not donate medications if they are within 6 months of their expiration date. However, each country and organization has its own policies on drug donation, and knowing the individual policy of the your host organization and visiting country is important. In addition, any donations should be appropriate to the diseases of the host country. Keep the medications in their appropriate containers to prevent any question about the identity of the medications and to get through customs with fewer hassles.

Most organizations can use and will welcome donations of almost any type of basic medical equipment or textbooks. However, you should be careful about donating medical equipment that will need ongoing maintenance, since these donations are often not sustainable or repairable if they break. For example, a piece of lab equipment or X-ray machine that needs special reagents or routine maintenance will soon be inoperable if there isn't money to support the maintenance. Bringing recent and up-to-date medical textbooks and journals is usually appreciated.

Here are some questions to ask:

- What medical equipment and supplies should I bring?
- What is the policy on drug donations?
- Are there specific supplies or books that I could bring as donations?
- What does it take to get my supplies and medication through customs?

Communications

Before departing, know the best way to communicate with people from home in case of an emergency or just to maintain regular contact. This is important from both ends, and will help prevent homesickness. Ask about the quality of phone service in the area where you will be working, and anticipate purchasing a local cell phone. Many countries have excellent cellular phone services that allow calls to the United States or Canada from even the most remote parts of the Amazon or sub-Saharan Africa. There are also satellite phones that will work even in the most remote areas of the world, but they may be rather expensive. Try to find out the cost of each option before you leave to avoid any big surprises when the bill arrives.

Also, having a calling card to use or using an Internet connection, such as Skype (www.skype.com), often facilitates communication and saves on cost. Internet services are becoming more frequent, but they may not be reliable in all countries. However, in most capital cities in hotels and Internet cafes, you will be able to send e-mail messages home. Finally, make sure you supply people at home with your contact information before your departure and send them updated information once you arrive (see the Personal Travel Form at the end of this chapter). Keep a written or electronic diary of your experience, including pictures with detailed descriptions. With digital cameras it is much easier to take hundreds of pictures and not worry about film or development until you return home. Consider setting up a blog so your friends, family, and supports can look into what you are doing or set up a group e-mail list to send them a note and some pictures on a regular basis.

Here are some questions to ask:

- What is the best way to communicate with people back home?
- Should I bring a laptop computer for Internet access?
- Should I plan to buy a cell phone after arriving?
- What is the contact information I can leave with people at home in case of an emergency?

Post-trip Debriefing

You should start to prepare for your return long before finishing your global health experience. First, consider whether you want or need to have some time off at home before starting back at work or school. Having about a week or 2 free after your return will not only help with jet lag, but will also give you some time to get your life back in order, and to minimize reverse culture shock. If you have been on a long-term assignment, then you may want some additional time to go to the dentist, get your financial affairs in order, visit with friends and relatives, set up living arrangements, etc. You may also want to make some time to thank the people and organization that has assisted you financially and logistically with your global health experience. However, if you don't want to lose any time upon your return, then you may want to arrange your rotation or work schedule early. Have your office or hospital know when you are returning to make sure you are on their schedule.

Finally, a few words of caution about the effects of 'reverse culture shock.' Yes, it is a real issue, and is most often experienced by people who are returning from their first long-term assignment. Those people who have been away for a long time will likely see their home environment in a new light. If returning from a resource-poor area to a resource-rich area, like Canada or the United States, these feelings often manifest in resentment of observed gluttony. 'They just don't know how good things are here,' is a common comment from people returning from a long-term assignment abroad. These feelings of reverse culture shock are common and should not be ignored. Talking about these feelings

with others who have had similar experiences can be extremely helpful.
Here are some questions to ask:

- Should I plan some time at home before restarting work or school?
- What do I need to do to reintegrate back into work or school?
- Am I experiencing 'reverse culture shock'?

List of Equipment

This is a suggested list of things you may want to bring, not what you
are required to bring. In general, people should attempt to travel as
lightly as possible. In addition, there may not be electricity available
where you are going, so consider your local environment when thinking of bringing anything that requires electricity. Remember that you
don't have to bring everything from home, and you can find most
things in nearby cities. As a general rule, don't bring anything that you
cannot afford to lose!

Travel

_____ Air mattress
_____ Backpack / suitcase
_____ Canteen / water bottle
_____ Cots
_____ Day pack (some travel backpacks have these attached!)
_____ Mosquito coils
_____ Mosquito net
_____ Mosquito repellent
_____ Pillow
_____ Sleeping bag / blankets
_____ Tent
_____ Water filter

*Clothing (Make sure you have appropriate clothing for the climate and
culture!)*

_____ Appropriate footwear (boots, shoes, sandals)
_____ Bras

_____ Contact lenses and sufficient cleaning fluid (bring a spare bottle)

_____ Dress / skirt

_____ Hat

_____ Jacket

_____ Long-sleeved dress shirts

_____ Raincoat / rainpants

_____ Shorts

_____ Slacks / jeans

_____ Socks

_____ Spare set of glasses (if you wear glasses)

_____ Sunglasses

_____ Sunscreen lotion

_____ Sweatshirt / sweatpants / sweaters

_____ Swimsuit

_____ T-shirts (may be donated at the end)

_____ Underwear (bring lots!)

_____ Warm clothes for cold weather

Personal

_____ Adaptors / converters (know what voltage you need)

_____ Bags (garbage bags to line suitcase to protect against rain especially during long bus rides!)

_____ Batteries (lots)

_____ Binoculars

_____ Books / textbooks

_____ Calculator

_____ Camera

_____ Candies / food

_____ Clothes pegs, scrub brush, laundry detergent

_____ Computer / computer files

_____ Condoms / contraceptives (Remember that abstinence is even safer)

_____ Cooking equipment

_____ Deodorant

_____ Elastic bands

_____ Feminine hygiene products

_____ Film / digital camera storage cards

_____ First aid kit

_____ Games (balloons, bubbles)

_____ Headlamp / flashlight

_____ Iodine tabs / water filter

_____ Lip balm

_____ Medical equipment (e.g., stethoscope)

_____ Money belt (but not a Fanny pack! – they are easily stolen)

_____ MP3 player / Walkman / radio

_____ Nail clippers

_____ Personal medications

_____ Pictures / postcards / books of your home country

_____ Pictures of your family

_____ Project materials

_____ Rope

_____ Sewing material / kit (with scissors)

_____ Shampoo

_____ Small mirror

_____ Soap

_____ Tape – duct, electrical

_____ Toilet paper / facial tissues

_____ Toiletries (toothbrush, toothpaste, dental floss, washcloth, comb, brush, hair elastics, barrettes)

_____ Towel (remember *The Hitchhiker's Guide to the Galaxy*!)

_____ Writing materials (journal / diary)

_____ Writing materials, paper, envelopes

Ask what you can buy where you're going, so that you don't bring too much!

Do *not* bring flashy jewellery or expensive watches!

Again, never bring anything that you cannot afford to lose!

Your Personal Travel Form

Personal	*Host contact*
Name:	Name:
Passport Information:	
Address:	Address:
Telephone / E-mail:	Telephone / E-mail:

Emergency Information

In case of emergency, contact (with telephone number):

Family Doctor (with telephone):

Pertinent Medical Problems

Personal Illnesses:

Current Medications (with dosages):

Allergies:

Travel and Flight Information

Flights

Date/Time: Date/Time:
Departure: Departure:
Arrival: Arrival:
Airline: Airline:
Flight No.:   Flight No.:

Date/Time: Date/Time:
Departure: Departure:
Arrival: Arrival:
Airline: Airline:
Flight No.:   Flight No.:

Travel Insurance

Name: Policy #:
Telephone:

Pertinent Particulars

Credit Card: Credit Card:
Telephone: Telephone:

Credit Card: Credit Card:
Telephone: Telephone:

Travellers Cheques

U.S. $20   Can $20

U.S. $50   Can $50

U.S. $100   Can $100

Recording Your Project

Name:
Address:

E-mail:
Faculty and Year:
Host Country:
Host Institution (contact names with address):

Faculty Adviser(s) (if any):

How did you prepare for it? (Include all resources – written, personal)

Costs involved:

Rating (on a scale of 1 to 10; 1= worst possible, 10 = the best project, highly recommended)

In one page or less, describe your activities. What you learned and what would make this project better.

International Opportunity Time Sheet

1 to 2 years before departure:
- Letters of inquiry for need or current program in place to area, country, or organization you are interested in
- Identify and engage funding sources
- Identify available time and duration

8 months before departure:
- Learn about medical needs, specific disease processes

- Identify and start to collect needed medical and pharmaceutical supplies
- Clearance for customs by host for supplies
- Apply for Continuing Medical Education credit
- Approval from appropriate person at work or school

6 months before departure:
- Fundraiser
- Language skills
- Identify housing, food services, and travel arrangements
- Receive country-specific immunizations
- Passport and visa application

3 months before departure:
- Contingency plan for last-minute changes
- Identify specific role, daily schedule

2 weeks before departure:
- Confirm all travel plans, accommodations, in-country travel
- Final packing and trip preparations
- Give family and friends communication information
- Start malaria prophylaxis if needed

1 month after return:
- Confirm all necessary requirements for credit
- Write thank-you and follow-up letters to your host
- Write a thank-you letter and a note outlining your trip to the school and to everyone that donated supplies, money, or assisted in any way
- Start making plans for the next trip!

Making Choices to Effect Change

Allan Rosenfield, MD
Dean, Mailman School of Public Health
Columbia University

Like my father, I trained to be an obstetrician and gynecologist and was fully prepared to enter into private medical practice in Boston. Before taking this path, however, I decided during my last year of residency to spend a year teaching at a new medical school in Lagos, Nigeria. I went to Africa with every expectation of returning in a year. Until then I had not given much thought to global health or demographic issues. This began to change thanks to a wonderful mentor at the teaching hospital in Nigeria, Dr Robert Wright, an internationally renowned public health expert. He was very interested in promoting family planning initiatives in Nigeria in order to give women choices about pregnancy and children. Personally, I began to consider broader health care issues in developing countries and the importance of being prevention-oriented with a focus on communities, rather than cure-oriented with a focus on the individual.

After my year in Nigeria, I took a job with the Population Council and was assigned to work in Thailand for a year. I thought I would certainly return to Boston after 1 more year, but I ended up staying in Thailand for 6 years. Working in Thailand as an adviser to the Ministry of Public Health was an extraordinary experience. I was fortunate to have started when the new undersecretary at the ministry decided to initiate a nationwide family planning program in response to Thailand's markedly high rate of population growth. At that time only physicians were allowed to prescribe contraceptive pills. However, there were far too few physicians in Thailand working in rural communities, as has been the situation in most developing countries. We conducted a small study to see if auxiliary midwives, working in small rural health facilities, could be trained to use a simple checklist and safely prescribe the pill. We demonstrated the expected results, and the ministry then authorized all auxiliary midwives to distribute the pill. This small act revolutionized the delivery of family planning services in Thailand, and the success of this program spread to many other countries.

Working in Nigeria and Thailand was a transformative experience that changed my life's trajectory. I witnessed populations with very high infant, child, and maternal mortality rates because of grossly inadequate health care services and systems. I realized that I could have a greater impact on the health of individuals by addressing the health needs of populations. Instead of returning to private practice in Boston, I chose to devote my career to some of the world's greatest public health challenges, including women's reproductive health, maternal mortality and morbidity, and the HIV/AIDS pandemic, which continues to devastate communities around the globe.

From my experiences, I've learned that working effectively in different cultures requires sensitivity and a willingness to adapt. One should develop an awareness of one's own attitudes, beliefs, and possible biases, as well as an understanding of the cultural norms and beliefs of the community. Always remain open to new ideas and different approaches to addressing health care issues. Do not assume that the Western medical system, with its high technological components, is necessarily the best model to follow in an underserved rural community. Become familiar with the conditions and constraints affecting people's lives, with a focus on the community's most vulnerable populations. Listen to and engage with people from different backgrounds, and appreciate the value of collaborating with others.

Taking the public health path was an important choice in my life, and one that has provided me with enormous professional and personal gratification. You will have many opportunities in your lives and will face many choices. You must find your own set of beliefs, and then seek out the opportunities to put your beliefs to work. From leaders in global health to those working at the front lines, everyone at some point has made choices to effect change. Some choices, even those that are seemingly insignificant, can turn out to have a major impact on your life and on the lives of others.

The Priority of Pandemics:
An Urgent Agenda in Global Health

Richard G.A. Feachem, CBE, FREng, DSc(Med), PhD
Professor of International Health
University of California at San Francisco and Berkeley
Former Executive Director of the Global Fund to Fight AIDS, Tuberculosis, and Malaria

The world faces a host of global challenges in the twenty-first century. Evidence is mounting for climate change having a potentially devastating social and economic impact. Recent terrorist attacks have raised the spectre of nuclear or chemical weapons falling into the hands of extremists, and the global powers struggle to confront this unconventional threat. The rapid growth of China and India has added to the global economy's already voracious appetite for natural resources and accentuated the need to develop alternative energy sources. The list continues. All of these global challenges are pressing, and all of them demand vigorous collective action by the global community.

The global community has finite financial and political resources available to tackle these challenges. So, in practice, we must prioritize them – a process that has become the focus of the annual summit of the Group of Eight nations. For two reasons, I believe that they and we should consistently place the challenge of global health pandemics at the top of the priority list.

The first reason is the massive global impact of these pandemics. HIV/AIDS continues to kill three million people every year and is bringing entire countries to their knees. Other infections such as malaria and tuberculosis kill millions more, fuelling the vicious cycle of poverty and thwarting efforts to close the gap between the global 'haves' and 'have nots.' The next pandemic of influenza, or perhaps a new pathogen, could easily cause hundreds of millions of deaths and cost trillions of dollars if we remain an unprepared global community.

The second reason for placing global health pandemics at the top of the global priorities list is that these goals cannot be achieved without concerted global effort. Two and a half decades of denial, ignorance, and inaction enabled HIV/AIDS to grow into the catastrophe it is today. Even the best prepared countries will be devastated by a major influenza pandemic if the rest of the world is not equally prepared.

Why do I tell you this? Because in the same way that the global community must decide how to prioritize its attention and resources, so must you as an individual. And so, just as I urge global leaders to commit their countries to the challenges of global health and pandemics, I urge you to do the same with your talents and energy.

There are massive opportunities for bright, committed people in the field of global health. Over the past 5 years the world has woken up to the need to and benefits of combatting infectious diseases and improving global health. We have demonstrated this by dramatically increasing the resources and political capital devoted to these issues. Key priorities, from rolling out treatment and prevention programs, to researching new technologies, to developing new policies and strategies, are now moving forward at an unprecedented speed. As a result, there is an insatiable appetite for manpower and a constantly growing need for people to translate new commitments and resources into lives saved and epidemics controlled.

You do not have to be a doctor or a molecular biologist to make a vital contribution to global health. Driving back the HIV/AIDS epidemic or preventing a new pandemic takes the full range of professional skills. Computer and technology specialists are needed to develop systems to plan and monitor programs. Lawyers and finance experts are needed to design and manage organizations that drive the global efforts. Writers and journalists are needed to attract and sustain the world's attention to critical health issues. These are only a few examples of how anyone can contribute to improving global health.

During my 40 years of working in health and development, and particularly during the past 5 years of launching and running a major international development finance institution, the Global Fund to Fight AIDS, Tuberculosis, and Malaria, I have come to realize that the single most important factor for determining whether health initiatives succeed or fail is the people who drive them. It was skilled and committed individuals who eradicated smallpox, one of the deadliest diseases humanity has ever faced. It has been determined individuals who have now driven polio to the brink of eradication. And so it could be you who helps eradicate malaria or tuberculosis or indeed, someday, HIV/AIDS. With millions of lives on the line each year, there are few ways to have a greater impact on the course of the world.

Making a Paradigm Shift: Global Health Delivery

Jim Kim, MD, PhD
Professor, Harvard Medical School
Founder, Partners in Health

Despite the many victories in global health over the past several years, there remains an enormous gap between what we know and what we have done about the world's most pressing health care problems. Millions of lives are lost every year from completely preventable or treatable diseases. These unnecessary deaths remind us of how much more work remains in delivering effective interventions to people living in resource-poor settings.

I have been fortunate over the course of my career to be a part of some extraordinary events in global health. When the non-governmental organization Partners in Health first encountered multidrug resistant tuberculosis (MDR-TB) in Haiti and Peru, the world's experts had already agreed that treating MDR-TB in poor communities was too expensive and too difficult. Rather than let these infections serve as a death sentence to the poor, we decided we had to treat our patients. What was the result? The result was exceptional cure rates that were better than in some U.S. hospitals. Today, in part because we proved that we could treat poor people, affordable treatment is now available for people suffering from MDR-TB around the world.

A recent World Health Organization program for HIV treatment, one in which I was closely involved, was the Initiative to Treat 3 Million People Living with HIV/AIDS by 2005, called '3 by 5.' Although we failed to reach our target, the initiative helped generate an enormous momentum for scaling up treatment with antiretroviral drugs. The number of HIV-infected people receiving treatment more than tripled, from 400,000 in mid-2003 to over 1.3 million at the end of 2005. Perhaps more significantly, there was an increase from 100,000 to 800,000 HIV-infected people receiving HIV medications in sub-Saharan Africa, which had been considered unreasonable just several years before this.

Throughout these experiences, the guiding principles of my work in global health have been social justice, equity, and a practical approach to addressing inequalities in access to health care. In reflecting on my more than two decades in global health, I believe that if we are serious about eliminating inequalities in health care, then we must begin by building a science of health care delivery in the world's poorest settings. For example, antiretroviral drugs can reduce mother-to-child transmission of HIV during pregnancy and breastfeeding by 40%. However, only 9% of all HIV-positive pregnant women and only 50% of pregnant women who test positive for HIV are provided with antiretroviral drugs. In addition, insecticide-treated bed nets used in malaria-endemic areas can reduce overall infant mortality by 30%, but only 3% of children in these regions are sleeping under bed nets. Furthermore, several new challenges in global health are starting to emerge, and they will bring even greater attention to our current shortcomings in health care delivery. The newly emerging threat of extensively drug-resistant tuberculosis (XDR-TB) could pose substantial public health problems in both developed and developing nations, especially for people infected with HIV.

Efforts to bridge gaps in health care delivery and to determine how to best provide quality health care for the world's poor and marginalized people presents one of the major challenges for the next generation of health care professionals. Harvard Medical School is currently working to develop an institute for global health delivery science in order to address this challenge. Through research in global health care delivery and direct efforts to improve implementation of health programs, the institute will work to transform our ability to deliver effective health interventions in resource-poor settings.

Compared with when I first began working in global health, the interest in global health and medicine has simply exploded. My generation has lived through both the lean times and the current 'golden age of global health.' We've learned much and even made some progress. When I meet all the remarkable young students, who are so committed to relieving the suffering of poor people throughout the world, I am encouraged and inspired beyond words.

A Call to Action for Global Health Education

Evaleen Jones, MD
Assistant Professor, Stanford University School of Medicine
Founder, Child Family Health International

> Never doubt that a small group of committed citizens can change the world. Indeed, it is the only thing that ever has.
> – Margaret Mead, U.S. anthropologist, 1901–1978

Medical School, 1988

I stormed out of the professor's office that afternoon, my cheeks streaked with tears of defiance. I had just returned from winter break and 5 weeks in Ecuador. Hoping to treat the increasing number of underserved, disenfranchised Spanish-speaking patients in our local emergency room and finding no formal student clerkships abroad, I had created a 'hand-tailored' overseas clinical rotation. After returning from Ecuador, I was convinced that every medical student should do the same: cross cultural and geographical borders, be challenged by the overwhelming health disparities in the developing world, question the extreme waste and excesses of the U.S. medical system, and discover a deeper appreciation for the luxuries we have at home. That day, my professor warned me that it was an impractical idea and an impossible dream. 'You have no experience in international health, no academic authority, and no idea of the issues and challenges of travelling abroad,' he said. 'You just can't do it.'

It was already too late. I had been 'bit by the bug,' and his comments were just the catalyst I needed to spark my passion and fuel my energy. Over the next two decades, I built the foundation for Child Family Health International (CFHI) to make similar experiences available to medical students like myself. In the words of Mark Twain, 'Travel is fatal to prejudice, bigotry and narrow-mindedness, and many of our people need it sorely on these accounts' (*Innocents Abroad*, published in 1869).

February 2008

In the last decade there has been a mind-boggling increase in the number of medical students and allied health professionals studying abroad. This growth calls for reflection and planning as we determine the moral and economic basis for global health education. We have the unique opportunity, if not obligation, to shepherd the globalization of health education with a human rights-based approach that is socially responsible and financially equitable.

We must continually challenge ourselves to question, examine, and judiciously evaluate the effectiveness and efficacy of overseas programs. Academic educators must continually seek to elevate the conscience of the medical institutions. Do we have the courage to design a framework that places research agendas on the back burner and makes the goals of our international partners the top priority? Can we create an educational model that mandates mutual benefit and holds to a standard of global sustainability?

International experiences expose people to unfamiliar situations that challenge them to reflect on their value system, examine their actions, and process difficult emotions. When challenged to live outside their comfort zone, students develop a new willingness for self-reflection and a deeper sense of humility. In addition, good mentoring can profoundly shape the leadership skills and professional identity of students. The passion and curiosity of young people is a major stimulant of moral action and public advocacy. Primum non nocere (First, do no harm) is a well-founded maxim taught in the medical community. Dr Delese Wear, Professor of Behavioural Sciences at Northeastern Ohio University, has suggested that we teach a new principle: Primum non tacere (Above all, do not keep silent).

I am optimistic that the changing nature of global health is adopting a stronger position on social justice. We also need to make medical education part of the solution to the global health crisis. Academic leaders must share two essential attributes with students: compassion and balance. Offering students the opportunity to practise sustained self-reflection and creating a safe environment for them to look boldly at their shortcomings nurtures humility. And, if we can demonstrate a healthy balance between our professional and personal lives, students will have a better chance to find fulfilment in their everyday activities. As the collective conscience of physicians grows stronger, the truths about the gross inequities and the physical limitations of our planet become more certain.

On a personal note, as a woman, a career path for women in global health before me had been largely unpaved. Recently, a medical student reflected that I seemed to have the 'perfect career' – teaching medical students, treating patients in a clinic, and publishing research, while maintaining a close and loving relationship with my family. I smiled inwardly. There's always another side to every story. What should I mention to her first? What should I leave out? In short, global health work has not always been easy and without sacrifice.

My advice is to be honest in your intentions, set realistic expectations, and be flexible in your plans. Seek and collect wise mentors, master acceptance, and follow your passion. Remember, all that you do is not all that you are. And the next time someone says you are too idealistic, unrealistic, inexperienced, unprepared, or ill equipped to follow your dreams, remember this:

> Those who say it cannot be done should not interrupt the person doing it.
> – Ancient Chinese Proverb

So, Go!

Keith Brown, MD
Assistant Professor,
University of Nebraska College of Medicine

Global health, international and remote medicine, what could be cooler? Travel to remote places, meet interesting people, and heal them! The dreams and expectations of dedicated, caring health care students and professionals all have a touch of Livingston, Schweitzer, and Clarke. But wait, there's more! Let's ground those dreams with a touch of reality and practicality, so that when you go forth to heal, you leave the rose-coloured glasses behind.

First, you'll be uncomfortable at times, physically, socially, and emotionally. Few places in the world are as consistently comfortable as day-to-day life in the United States. Too hot, too cold, too wet, too dry, too windy, too dusty, too many bugs – *that's* the reality of much of the world. The social environment, however, can be an even larger stressor. No matter how welcoming and friendly your hosts and your patients are – and they will be – small differences can make for big culture shock. Simple mannerisms may mean something different or even be quite rude. Jokes fall flat. Assumptions about behavioural norms seem to be consistently wrong. This enhances the sense of isolation and emotional stress that you *will* experience. Missing family and friends, comfort foods, and 'normal' activities, all this is all 'normal' and you should anticipate it.

Know that you'll have to make sacrifices. Global health work requires money, time, family understanding, and making priorities in your life. It's expensive to travel, and even living in very simple conditions can cost quite a bit. You can get by with much less than you think you can, but it requires experience to learn this. Time away from school and work is always an issue. Even as a scheduled rotation, the time away can be difficult depending on what resources you have available to manage things while you are gone, not to mention returning exhausted and jumping right back into things. Family needs can be tough. Leaving a spouse and/or children behind for a remote location, where you may have little or no communications, can be a terrible stressor. All of these issues and more mean that you really must want to do global health work. Don't underestimate the sacrifices.

Be ready for *everyone* to tell you why going overseas is a bad idea, whether they be spouses, friends, parents, classmates, or teachers. Everyone will have a reason why it's a bad idea. It's not safe. Everyone hates Americans. It's too expensive. You'll be gone too long. You won't study enough for boards. You won't be able to help when great Uncle Bob paints his house – you name it, someone will offer it up as a reason not to go. Well, this becomes part of making sacrifices, doesn't it? You may have to take some grief from those you care about. You may have to make some people mad, or disappoint someone. You may miss some important dates. Only you can decide if the benefits are worth the costs.

Finally, understand why you are there: you are there for *you*. All of us who have worked in global health have done so out of a desire to help, to make a difference, to *do good*. Well, to *do good*, to make a difference, you have to be present for very long periods of time, like years. Short-term medical projects and rotations are extremely helpful – *for those who participate in them*. You will have the opportunity to experience medicine – and life – as you may never have before. You will be exposed to attitudes, assumptions, prejudices, and ideas you never even considered possible. You will experience a completely new facet of the human condition, good and bad. And that's why the project or rotation is for you. Yes, you'll make some diagnoses, curse some acute conditions, and plant some educational seeds. But to make a real difference for patients, for their community – that requires building an infrastructure of public health, public education, and a million other things that aren't in the medical curriculum. Don't feel guilty or regretful about not 'doing good.' The good will come, in the entire rest of your career and in the countless patients who will benefit from you being a better, more humane medical professional.

So, what? So, go! Go, knowing that in return for a comparatively small effort on your part, the patients you will be seeing and living with will reward you with everything that they have. And that *you* will get the better part of the deal.

10 Conclusions and 25 Pearls for Global Health

Global health and medicine are exciting ways to see the world while improving the health of people in less-developed regions. The greatest difficulty that most people have usually is not in deciding to embark on some international experience, but in determining how to get started. A variety of global health topics and issues have been covered in this guidebook. Hopefully, these chapters have given the sense that becoming engaged in global health is both possible and realistic. Since global health encompasses a wide range of backgrounds and experiences, nobody should be deterred. Finding a suitable position may take some effort, but is almost always well worth the investment. Furthermore, one global health experience often leads to another, and several doors are typically available for a subsequent global health experience.

Many people have altruistic impressions of those working in global health and medicine. While working to improve the health of people in developing countries is a privilege and can be very rewarding, it can also provide for a very nice lifestyle. Developing relationships with people from another culture can be enriching, on many levels, and typically the decreased cost of living can allow for more domestic support. Some combination of these characteristics, as well as others, often builds a sense of commitment to conducting global health work in developing countries. In this way, some people can explore their interests and find their passions in global health and medicine. We encourage you to explore your interests and discover your passions in global health and medicine.

Global Health Pearls

This final section lists some recommendations, or pearls, for any global health experience. They have been developed through our experiences, both successes and failures, and evolved through conversations with other global health experts. This list is by no means fully inclusive of all relevant suggestions. However, they are our favourites.

1 *Believe you can make a difference.* Any person can have a lasting effect of improving the lives of people around the world. You have to believe that your efforts can make a difference before you can even get started.
2 *Find good mentors.* A good mentor can open doors and opportunities that you may have never realized even existed. Along the same lines, *be* a good mentor when others start asking you for advice.
3 *Become involved with organizations that interest you.* Not every global health organization is going to be suited to your interests and goals, so become active with organizations that share your interests and goals.
4 *Nothing replaces experience.* The more one experiences working in global health, the more one can contribute to helping others in different locations.
5 *Don't let funding be your obstacle.* This is often considered to be a great inhibitor of global health experiences, but it shouldn't be. Asking local religious organizations and community clubs and seeking out various grants should make it easy to do global health work.
6 *Prepare yourself before departure.* Orienting to the location, language, culture, and customs of the community that you will be working in is extremely important. Acquiring as much of this knowledge as possible before leaving is paramount.
7 *Don't take things you can't afford to lose.* While travelling, things get lost all the time. If you think something is too valuable to lose, then leave it at home.
8 *Experience the culture.* It is often easy to blend into expatriate communities abroad. By experiencing the culture, you will learn more about the difficulties faced by the local communities. There is nothing like actually hauling a few gallons of water with the local children.
9 *Be respectful.* Do not do anything abroad that you would not do at home. Remember, global health experiences are a privilege, not a right.

10 *Know your limitations.* Do not try to work out of your range of skills. This is not the place to practise some new surgical procedure, for instance.

11 *Be invited.* So often, there is a paternalistic attitude towards working in global health. One of the key methods to avoid imposing is to offer your help. If your offer is rejected, then it probably would not have been used anyway.

12 *Build partnerships.* Global health involves a broad coalition of partners, so be prepared to build those partnerships.

13 *Learn from overseas colleagues.* One of the most important things for being effective is to actively listen. Colleagues overseas are very good at articulating their needs and wishes. Sometimes, all you have to do is listen.

14 *Set specific and realistic goals.* Understand what you can accomplish given your resources and time, and then set realistic goals.

15 *Inform your overseas colleagues.* All too often, the results of projects and work are not shared with the local communities. However, we have an obligation to tell the overseas colleagues or communities about our findings and to help them achieve improvements.

16 *Think long term.* Even if you are going for only a few weeks, work with projects that have commitments to support the sustainable development of local communities.

17 *Your priorities are second.* Your first priority is to address the needs of the local community.

18 *Monitor and evaluate your impact.* Be frank and honest with yourself and your colleagues about what has and has not worked well with your activities or projects, and then be prepared to modify them.

19 *Learn from the mistakes of others.* Look for ways to improve current programs, and learn to recognize why some previous programs have failed to achieve their goals.

20 *Take care of yourself.* Never take your own health for granted. Visit a travel clinic before departure. Wear sunscreen and avoid infectious diseases. If you are not feeling well, then take time to heal yourself. You will be of little help to others until you do.

21 *Wear your seatbelt.* The number one killer of overseas development workers is not infectious disease, but motor vehicle accidents. Not wearing a seatbelt or sitting on the back of an open-bed truck is dangerous, particularly on poorly maintained or unpaved roads.

22 *Remember your family and loved ones.* Sharing photos about your family from home is a great way to build rapport. If you want to partic-

ipate in global health in the long run, then you should incorporate your family and loved ones into your global health experiences.

23 *Become an activist.* Global health needs both national and international advocates. Learn to influence others on global health issues, particularly after you have some relevant global health experience.

24 *Share your stories.* Working in a developing country is a unique experience. Synthesize what you're learned, and inform others who may be interested in global health. Continuing to expand the impact of global health will require more people and more awareness.

25 *Have fun!* Global health work can be an exciting and highly rewarding experience.

Appendix: Additional Global Health Resources

Many additional global health resources are available for those seeking more information. The resources presented in this chapter are organized by the following categories: books, journal articles, annual reports, medical and public health journals, and videos and documentaries.

Books

Achebe C. *Things Fall Apart*. London: Anchor Books, 1994.

Basch PF. *Vaccines and World Health: Science, Policy, and Practice*. Oxford: Oxford University Press, 1994.

Basch PF. *Textbook of International Health*, 2nd ed. Oxford: Oxford University Press, 1999.

Beaglehole R (ed). *Global Public Health: A New Era*. Oxford: Oxford University Press, 2003.

Birrell K, Birrell G. *Diagnosis and Treatment: A Training Manual for Primary Health Care Workers*. London: Macmillan, 2000.

Black M. *The No-Nonsense Guide to International Development*. London: Verso, 2002.

Boelart M, et al. *Nutritional Guidelines*. Paris: Médecins sans Frontières, 1995.

Brabazon J. *Albert Schweitzer: A Biography*, 2nd ed. Syracuse: Syracuse University Press, 2000.

Bryant J. *Health in the Developing World*. Ithaca: Cornell University Press, 1969.

Burns AA, Lovich R, Maxwell J, Shapiro K. *Where Women Have No Doctor*. Berkeley: Hesparian Foundation, 2002.

Desjarlais R, Eisenberg L, Good B, Kleinman A. *World Mental Health:*

Problems and Priorities in Low-Income Countries. Oxford: Oxford University Press, 1995.

Edleston M, Pierini S. *Oxford Handbook of Tropical Medicine.* Oxford: Oxford University Press, 2002.

Fadiman A. *The Spirit Catches You and You Fall Down.* New York: Farrar, Straus and Giroux, 1998.

Farmer P. *Infections and Inequalities.* Berkeley: University of California Press, 1999.

Farmer P. *Pathologies of Power: Health, Human Rights, and the New War on the Poor.* Berkeley: University of California Press, 2003.

Fink S. *War Hospital: A True Story of Surgery and Survival.* New York: Public Affairs, 2003.

Fisher J. *Non Governments: NGOs and the Political Development of the Third World.* Sterling, VA: Kumarian Press, 1998.

Garrett L. *The Coming Plague: Newly Emerging Diseases in a World Out of Balance.* New York: Farrar, 1994.

Garrett L. *Betrayal of Trust: The Collapse of Global Public Health.* New York: Hyperion, 2000.

Gourevitch P. *We Wish to Inform You that Tomorrow We Will Be Killed with Our Families: Stories from Rwanda.* New York: Picador, 1999.

Hilts P. *Rx for Survival: Why We Must Rise to the Global Health Challenge.* New York: Penguin, 2005.

Honigsbaum M. *The Fever Trail: In Search of the Cure for Malaria.* New York: Farrar, Straus and Giroux, 2001.

Jong E, McMullen R. *The Travel and Tropical Medicine Handbook*, 3rd ed. Philadelphia: WB Saunders, 2002.

Kapuscinski R. *The Shadow of the Sun.* Toronto: Vintage, 2002.

Kasmauski K, Jaret P. *Impact: On the Frontlines of Global Health.* Washington, DC: National Geographic Press, 2003.

Kaul I, Grunberg I, Stern MA. *Global Public Goods.* Oxford: Oxford University Press, 1999.

Kidder T. *Mountain beyond Mountains: Healing the World – The Quest of Dr Paul Farmer.* New York: Random House, 2003.

Kim JY, Millen JV, Irwin A, Gershman J (eds). *Dying for Growth: Global Inequality and the Health of the Poor.* Monroe: Common Courage Press, 2000.

Koop CE, Pearson CE, Schwarz MR (eds). *Critical Issues in Global Health.* San Francisco: Jossey-Bass, 2001.

Kopolow D. *Smallpox: The Fight to Eradicate a Global Scourge.* Berkeley: University of California Press, 2003.

Lankester T. *Setting Up Community Health Programmes: A Practical Manual for Use in Developing Countries*, 2nd ed. London: Macmillan, 2000.

Leaning J, Briggs SM, Chen LC (eds). *Humanitarian Crises: The Medical and Public Health Response*. Cambridge: Harvard University Press, 1999.

Levine R. *Millions Saved: Proven Successes in Global Health*. Washington, DC: Center for Global Development, 2004.

Levine R. *Case Studies in Global Health: Millions Saved*. Sudbury, MA: Jones and Bartlett, 2007.

Lindstrand A, Bergström S, Rosling H, Rubenson B, Stenson B. *Global Health: An Introductory Textbook*. Lund: Studentlitteratur, 2006.

Loos GP. *Field Guide for International Health Project Planners and Managers*. London: Janus, 1996.

Mann JM, Gruskin S, Grodin MA, Annas GJ (eds). *Health and Human Rights: A Reader*. New York: Routledge, 1999.

Maphorogo S, Sutter E [Jenkins J (ed)]. *The Community Is My University: A Voice from the Grass Roots on Rural Health and Development*. Amsterdam: KIT, 2004.

McKee M, Garner P, Stott R (eds). *International Co-operation in Health*. Oxford: Oxford University Press, 2001.

Médecins sans Frontières. *Quiet, We Are Dying. Testimonies, An Excerpt from Meurt, Democratic Republic of Congo*. www.msf.ca/drc/quiet.pdf

Merson MH, Black RE, Mills AJ (eds). *International Public Health: Diseases, Programs, Systems and Policies*, 2nd ed. Gaithersburg: Aspen, 2005.

Noji EK (ed). *The Public Health Consequences of Disasters*. Oxford: Oxford University Press, 1997.

O'Neil Jr E. *Awakening Hippocrates: A Primer on Health, Poverty, and Global Service*. Washington, DC: American Medical Association, 2006.

O'Neil Jr E. *A Practical Guide to Global Health Service*. Washington, DC: American Medical Association, 2006.

Osborn G, Ohmans P. *Finding Work in Global Health: A Practical Guide for Job Seekers or Anyone Who Wants to Make the World a Healthier Place*. Saint Paul: Health Advocates Press, 2005.

Rohde J, Wyon J (eds). *Community-Based Health Care: Lessons from Bangladesh to Boston*. Boston: Management Sciences for Health, 2002.

Sachs J. *The End of Poverty: Economic Possibilities for Our Time*. New York: Penguin, 2005.

Schull RC. *Common Medical Problems in the Tropics*, 2nd ed. London: Macmillan, 1999.

Schweitzer A, Antje Bultman L, Cart J, Miller RS. *Out of My Life and Thought: An Autobiography.* Baltimore: Johns Hopkins University Press, 1998.

Sen A. *Development as Freedom.* New York: Anchor, 2000.

Sidel V, Levy B (eds). *War and Public Health.* New York: Oxford University Press, 1997.

Skolnik, R. *Essentials of Global Health.* Sudbury, MA: Jones and Bartlett, 2007.

Stanfield P, Balldin B, Versluys Z. *Child Health: A Manual for Medical and Health Workers in Health Centres and Rural Health*, 2nd ed. Nairobi: African Medical and Research Foundation, 1997.

Werner D. *Disabled Village Children.* Palo Alto: Hesperian Foundation, 1988.

Werner D, Bower B. *Helping Health Workers Learn.* Palo Alto: Hesperian Foundation, 1992.

Werner D, Sanders D. *Questioning the Solution: The Politics of Primary Health Care and Child Survival.* Palo Alto: HealthWrights, 1996.

Werner D, Thuman C, Maxwell J. *Where There Is No Doctor: A Village Health Care Handbook.* Palo Alto: Hesperian Foundation, 2004.

Whitney RL. *Slim.* College Station: Texas A&M University Press, 2003.

Williams WC. *The Doctor Stories.* New York: New Directions Publishing Company, 1984.

Journal Articles

Journal articles can be found for almost any topic or issue in global health and medicine. The best place to search for published journal articles is through PubMed (www.pubmed.gov), an international journal database maintained by the National Library of Medicine. An additional bibliography of over 870 global health articles can be found at the Global Health Education Consortium website (www.globalhealth-ec. org/GHEC/Resources/Ghbiblio_resources.htm). The site is regularly edited and maintained by Kevin Chan at the University of Toronto and by Jessie Evert and Tom Hall at the University of California at San Francisco.

Annual Reports

Many of the large multinational organizations that conduct work related to global health and medicine produce annual reports. A listing of these organizations with the website to their annual report is provided below.

Joint U.N. Program on HIV/AIDS
Title: Annual Epidemic Update
Website: www.unaids.org

U.N. Development Program
Title: Annual Reports on Human Development
Website: hdr.undp.org

UNICEF
Title: State of the World's Children
Website: www.unicef.org

World Bank
Title: World Development Report
Website: www.worldbank.org/wdr

World Health Organization
Title: The World Health Report
Website: www.who.int/whr/en/

Medical and Public Health Journals

Several medical and public health journals devote all or part of their content to relevant global health issues. Some of the more prominent journals covering global health and their websites are provided below.

AIDS
www.aidsonline.com

American Journal of Public Health
www.ajph.org

American Journal of Tropical Medicine and Hygiene
www.ajtmh.org

British Medical Journal
www.bmj.com

Bulletin of the World Health Organization
www.who.int/bulletin/en/

Canadian Medical Association Journal
www.cmaj.ca

Global Public Health
www.tandf.co.uk/journals/titles/17441692.asp

Global Pulse
www.amsa.org/globalpulse

Lancet
www.thelancet.com

New England Journal of Medicine
content.nejm.org

Population and Development Review
www.blackwellpublishing.com/pdr

Science
www.sciencemag.org

Social Science and Medicine
www.elsevier.com/wps/find/journaldescription.cws_home/315/
description#description

Tropical Medicine and International Health
www.blackwellpublishing.com/journals/tmi/

Videos and Documentaries

Here are a few of the documentaries devoted specifically to global
health issues and topics.

A Closer Walk, New Version (85 min). Worldwide Documentaries. 2006–7.
China Blue. Teddy Bear Films. www.teddybearfilms.com/. 2006
Darwin's Nightmare. Celluloid Dreams. www.darwinsnightmare.com.
  2004.
Faces of AIDS in Mozambique (6 min) and *Treatment for Life: Sofia's Story*
  (16 min). Health Alliance International. depts.washington.edu/
  haiuw. 2005.
Haba Na Haba (Little by Little). Casade Health Communications Group.
  depts.washington.edu/healthy. 2003.
Hold Your Breath. Program in Bioethics and Film, Stanford University.
  www.medethicsfilms.stanford.edu. 2005.

Invisible Children: Discover the Unseen. Invisible Children. www. invisiblechildren.com

Rx for Survival – A Global Health Challenge. WGBH Educational Foundation and Vulcan Productions Inc. 2005.

Salud! (93 min). Bourne, Field, Keck and Reed. MEDICC. www.saludthefilm.net. 2006.

Silent Killer: The Unfinished Campaign against Hunger. KCTS Television. www.silentkillerfilm.org. 2005.

Unnatural Causes: Is Inequality Making Us Sick? California Newsreel. www.unnaturalcauses.org. 2008.

Worlds Apart: A Four-Part Series on Cross Cultural Health Care. Program in Bioethics and Film, Stanford University. www.medethicsfilms. stanford.edu/. 2003.

Web Resources

Several recent web-based free-access teaching modules review pertinent global health issues, including those on the following list.

Global Health Education Consortium. 'Global Health Course Modules Project.' San Francisco, 2007. www.globalhealth-ec.org/GHEC/ Home/Modules.htm

Kaiser Family Foundation. 'Global Health Reporting.' Menlo Park, 2008. globalhealthreporting.org

Stanford University. 'Rethinking International Health.' Palo Alto, 2007. rih.stanford.edu

U.S. Agency for International Development. 'Global Health eLearning Center.' Washington, DC. www.globalhealthlearning.org/login.cfm

Index